D0108780

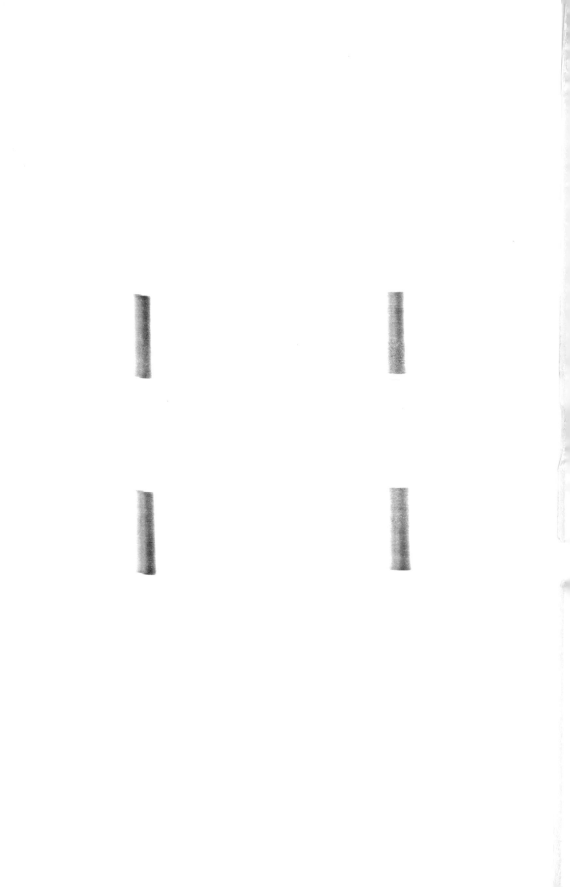

What You Need to Know about Headaches

What You Need to Know about Headaches

Claudio Butticè

Inside Diseases and Disorders

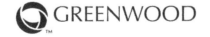 GREENWOOD

An Imprint of ABC-CLIO, LLC

Santa Barbara, California • Denver, Colorado

Copyright © 2022 by ABC-CLIO, LLC

All rights reserved. No part of this publication may be reproduced, stored in a retrieval system, or transmitted, in any form or by any means, electronic, mechanical, photocopying, recording, or otherwise, except for the inclusion of brief quotations in a review, without prior permission in writing from the publisher.

This book discusses treatments (including types of medication and mental health therapies), diagnostic tests for various symptoms and mental health disorders, and organizations. The authors have made every effort to present accurate and up-to-date information. However, the information in this book is not intended to recommend or endorse particular treatments or organizations, or substitute for the care or medical advice of a qualified health professional, or be used to alter any medical therapy without a medical doctor's advice. Specific situations may require specific therapeutic approaches not included in this book. For those reasons, we recommend that readers follow the advice of qualified health care professionals directly involved in their care. Readers who suspect they may have specific medical problems should consult a physician about any suggestions made in this book.

Library of Congress Cataloging-in-Publication Data

Names: Butticè, Claudio, author.
Title: What you need to know about headaches / Claudio Butticè.
Description: Santa Barbara, California : Greenwood, [2022] | Series: Inside
  diseases and disorders | Includes bibliographical references and index.
Identifiers: LCCN 2021030477 (print) | LCCN 2021030478 (ebook) | ISBN
  9781440875311 (hardcover) | ISBN 9781440875328 (ebook)
Subjects: LCSH: Headache.
Classification: LCC RC392 .B83 2022 (print) | LCC RC392 (ebook) | DDC
  616.8/491—dc23
LC record available at https://lccn.loc.gov/2021030477
LC ebook record available at https://lccn.loc.gov/2021030478

ISBN: 978-1-4408-7531-1 (print)
      978-1-4408-7532-8 (ebook)

26 25 24 23 22 1 2 3 4 5

This book is also available as an eBook.

Greenwood
An Imprint of ABC-CLIO, LLC

ABC-CLIO, LLC
147 Castilian Drive
Santa Barbara, California 93117
www.abc-clio.com

This book is printed on acid-free paper ∞

Manufactured in the United States of America

To all those people who, like me, must survive with a demon that once in a while (and always one time too many) tries to claw out of their heads, leaving a trail of destruction in its wake. Even when the pain seems unbearable, hold tight. It will always fade away—eventually.

Contents

CHAPTER 8
Prevention *107*

CHAPTER 9
Issues and Controversies *119*

CHAPTER 10
Current Research and Future Directions *129*

Series Foreword

Disease is as old as humanity itself, and it has been the leading cause of death and disability throughout history. From the Black Death in the Middle Ages to smallpox outbreaks among Native Americans to the modern-day epidemics of diabetes and heart disease, humans have lived with—and died from—all manner of ailments, whether caused by infectious agents, environmental and lifestyle factors, or genetic abnormalities. The field of medicine has been driven forward by our desire to combat and prevent disease and to improve the lives of those living with debilitating disorders. And while we have made great strides forward, particularly in the last 100 years, it is doubtful that mankind will ever be completely free of the burden of disease.

Greenwood's Inside Diseases and Disorders series examines some of the key diseases and disorders, both physical and psychological, affecting the world today. Some (such as diabetes, cardiovascular disease, and ADHD) have been selected because of their prominence within modern America. Others (such as Ebola, celiac disease, and autism) have been chosen because they are often discussed in the media and, in some cases, are controversial or the subject of scientific or cultural debate.

Because this series covers so many different diseases and disorders, we have striven to create uniformity across all books. To maximize clarity and consistency, each book in the series follows the same format. Each begins with a collection of 10 frequently asked questions about the disease or disorder, followed by clear, concise answers. Chapter 1 provides a general introduction to the disease or disorder, including statistical information such as prevalence rates and demographic trends. The history of the disease or disorder, including how our understanding of it has evolved over time, is addressed in chapter 2. Chapter 3 examines causes and risk factors, whether genetic, microbial, or environmental, while chapter 4 discusses signs and symptoms. Chapter 5 covers the issues of diagnosis (and misdiagnosis), treatment, and management (whether with drugs, medical procedures, or lifestyle changes). How such treatment, or the lack thereof, affects a patient's long-term prognosis, as well as the risk of complications, are the subject of chapter 6. Chapter 7 explores the disease or disorder's effects on the friends and family of a patient—a dimension often overlooked in discussions of physical and psychological ailments. Chapter 8 discusses prevention strategies, while chapter 9 explores key issues or controversies, whether medical or sociocultural. Finally, chapter 10 profiles cutting-edge research and speculates on how things might change in the next few decades.

Each volume also features five fictional case studies to illustrate different aspects of the book's subject matter, highlighting key concepts and themes that have been explored throughout the text. The reader will also find a glossary of terms and a collection of print and electronic resources for additional information and further study.

As a final caveat, please be aware that the information presented in these books is no substitute for consultation with a licensed health care professional. These books do not claim to provide medical advice or guidance.

Introduction

His headache was still sitting over his right eye as if it had been nailed there.

—Ian Fleming

Every one of us has had to deal with a headache at least once. Headaches can affect anyone, regardless of race, gender, age, or preexisting conditions. According to the World Health Organization (WHO), nearly 50% of adults across the world will experience a headache in any given year.

Headaches can be caused by external factors such as stress, medical conditions, or toxic substances, or they can just become a condition on their own. Although a headache is most often a symptom of something else, many headaches can become real disorders with a significant impact on the quality of life of those affected. Depending on the severity and frequency, a headache may range from a mildly annoying issue to a truly debilitating and disabling condition that negatively affects the entire existence of a person.

A headache may hit at any time, and when it does, there are very few other things you can think about other than getting rid of it as quickly as possible. They often lead to other problems, as they are linked with several comorbidities such as depression, anxiety, and mood disorders. They're associated with social stigma and may represent a huge health burden when they become frequent or chronic. People suffering from frequent migraines, for example, may have serious issues attending school or work regularly. Headache disorders are not just an individual health and economic burden for those affected. They are among the leading causes of years lived with disability (YLD) worldwide and have a tremendous impact on society at large. Even famous historic figures such as Charles Darwin, Julius Caesar, Sigmund Freud, Thomas Jefferson, and Napoleon suffered from debilitating headaches that forced them to endure tremendous pain and, in some instances, led to their withdrawal from society.

It is probably impossible to thoroughly describe how taxing the weight of such a condition can be on the physical and emotional balance of a person. The purpose of this book is to educate the public about headaches in general, their broad effects on the lives of those affected, their social and economic impact, and much more. More than anything else, what we're striving for is showing our readers the world from the perspective of people with a significant headache disorder.

It is important to note how most scientific literature on headaches centers on migraine, and thus, much of the data pertaining to headaches that are cited throughout this book can only refer to this condition. However, much of this information, especially when it comes to quality-of-life aspects, psychosocial consequences, and overall burden of the disease, is overlapping or at least easily comparable with the other, less-studied primary headache disorders. Because of that, we will interchangeably make use of terms such as "severe headaches" or "major headaches" to include, in a broader sense, those headaches that significantly affect the life of sufferers—namely, trigeminal autonomic cephalalgias (paroxysmal hemicrania, hemicrania continua, cluster headache, and SUNCT/SUNA), trigeminal neuralgia, chronic tension-type headache, and all those primary and secondary headaches that severely hamper the lives of sufferers because of their frequency or severity.

Essential Questions

1. HOW CAN I TELL THAT MY HEADACHE IS NOT A BRAIN TUMOR?

Although headaches are a main symptom of many brain tumors, most headaches are not related to cerebral neoplasia. Headaches caused by tumors are usually quite different from the other headaches you have suffered during your life. This very difference, together with the sudden onset, is usually a first warning sign that something is wrong and that you need to seek your doctor's advice. Headaches caused by tumors are generally very severe, tend to be worse in the morning, and may wake you up at night. They're also associated with nausea and vomiting and do not respond to most over-the-counter medications. However, these symptoms alone are not sufficient for a brain tumor diagnosis, as they are associated with several other types of primary or secondary headache disorders as well.

2. CAN MY LIFESTYLE AND DIET AFFECT THE FREQUENCY OF MY HEADACHE ATTACKS?

Several lifestyle changes, including establishing consistent sleep hygiene practices, healthy dietary habits, and proper physical exercise routines, can positively affect the quality of life of patients affected by many primary headache disorders. Many patients who follow some simple rules to develop positive lifestyle habits experience a reduction in the number of headache attacks as well as the severity of each episode. Similarly, quitting many unhealthy lifestyle habits, such as limiting the consumption of alcohol or junk food, stopping or reducing cigarette smoking or tobacco use, or moving away from a sedentary lifestyle may also have a positive impact on migraine and other headache disorders.

3. ARE HEADACHES DANGEROUS OR LIFE-THREATENING?

Most primary headaches are not inherently dangerous or life-threatening conditions, although they may significantly lower the quality of life of the patient. Some comorbid conditions are, however, associated with poor health outcomes such as depression, anxiety, and substance abuse and may, in rare instances, lead to suicide. On the other hand, a minority of secondary headaches may signal a potentially lethal underlying condition. Some dangerous conditions, such as brain tumors, intracranial hemorrhages, and cerebral venous thrombosis, have a side effect of headaches and must be promptly identified to ensure that they are treated quickly and effectively.

4. HOW PAINFUL CAN A HEADACHE ATTACK BE?

The severity of the pain of a headache mostly depends on the type of disorder affecting the sufferer. With some headache disorders, such as tension-type headaches, the pain is generally mild to moderate, but it may last for many hours. Other headache disorders, such as cluster headache or paroxysmal hemicrania, are instead characterized by searing, excruciating pain. This unique form of agonizing pain is ranked among the most painful experiences known to medicine, including amputations, childbirth, and breakthrough cancer pain.

5. IS IT POSSIBLE FOR ONE PERSON TO HAVE SEVERAL TYPES OF HEADACHES?

It is possible, and potentially even really common, to suffer from multiple types of headaches at the same time. People affected by a long-term primary headache disorder, such as migraine, may also suffer from some secondary headache disorder at some point during their lives. For example, they may suffer a head injury and develop an acute or persistent post-traumatic headache. However, people with severe or chronic primary headache disorders such as migraine, cluster headache, and paroxysmal hemicrania are more likely to suffer from a comorbidity with other primary headache disorders. It is hard to tell whether this comorbidity may simply be attributed to an initial uncommon clinical presentation due to the high risk of misdiagnosis associated with these diseases.

6. IS IT POSSIBLE TO "CURE" OR OUTGROW A HEADACHE OR MIGRAINE FOREVER?

It is technically possible to "cure" many secondary headaches if the underlying condition that causes them (e.g., a head trauma or a vascular malformation) is resolved. For most primary headaches and migraines, however, a cure is not yet available, but attacks can be prevented and reduced in number and intensity by a significant margin. Also, migraine and some trigeminal autonomic cephalalgias generally improve as a patient gets older than 50 or 60 years of age. Up to 40% of migraine patients stop having attacks by the age of 65. Nonetheless, although there's a chance of outgrowing one's headache disorder, there are many unfortunate people who still suffer from these conditions in their sixties, seventies, and eighties.

7. DOES COFFEE TRIGGER OR TREAT HEADACHES?

Some people with headaches report that strong coffee can abort or provide relief during an attack, while others claim that it can act as a trigger, so what's the truth? Caffeine can actually help treat some tension-type headaches and, in some instances, even migraine, for several reasons: First, it may aid in the body's absorption of several medications, especially acetaminophen and other pain relievers, and increase their effects. Second, caffeine has a vasoconstrictive property that counteracts the vasodilation typically associated with headache pain. However, although with occasional use it may provide modest acute headache relief, too much of the substance can trigger tolerance and dependency, reducing its effectiveness over time. Eventually, caffeine dependency may also cause rebound headaches during withdrawal periods.

8. HOW CAN I TELL THE DIFFERENCE BETWEEN A COMMON HEADACHE AND A MIGRAINE?

The biggest difference between a migraine and a common headache lies in its severity and associated disability. A migraine episode is always highly disabling and will force a sufferer to stay put for several hours. Any attempt to "push through" it will only make things significantly worse. Migraines are also associated with several neurological and physical symptoms, mostly strong nausea and/or vomiting, vision disturbances, hypersensitivity to sounds or smells, and general prostration.

9. ARE PEOPLE WITH MIGRAINES OR FREQUENT HEADACHES MORE INTELLIGENT THAN NONSUFFERERS?

Since many famous historical figures such as Napoleon or Julius Caesar suffered from excruciating or recurrent headaches, it is a common myth that people with migraine are more intelligent. However, recent studies that examined the prevalence of migraine in different individuals debunked this false belief. In fact, there's no credible evidence that individuals with migraine are more intelligent or of higher social class. What is true, on the other hand, is that more-intelligent individuals affected by migraine, and more generally, those in higher social classes, are more likely to consult a doctor for their headaches.

10. CAN CHILDREN GET MIGRAINES?

Sadly, childhood migraine is a highly disabling condition that can seriously affect the child's quality of life. Kids and teens tend to develop anticipatory anxiety, which may disrupt their lives even further. However, the clinical presentation of migraine is somewhat different in children compared with adults—namely, attacks are shorter and less frequent—making it difficult to diagnose it and provide effective treatment. Between 7.7% and 9.1% of school-age children suffer from migraine, and the statistic may rise to up to 28% during adolescence (15–19 years of age). Children with at least one parent with migraine have a 50% chance of inheriting it, and that chance increases to 75% if both parents suffer from this condition.

1

What Are Headaches?

*Headaches were like birds. Starlings. They could be per-
fectly calm, then a single acorn could drop and send the
entire flock to the sky.*

—Erika Swyler

There are nearly 200 different types of headaches—each one is a very different and peculiar condition. *The International Classification of Headache Disorders*, third edition (*ICHD*-3), lists all that matters about each of
them (symptoms, pathogenesis, etiology, etc.) in an incredibly detailed
way. Since the introduction of this classification, in less than 30 years,
headache grew from one of the worst-classified neurological diseases to
the best-classified one. Today, no other neurology subspecialty has such a
systematic classification in neurological diseases. However, despite this
incredible level of detail, the true mechanisms behind the many headache
disorders still remain a mystery deeply buried inside the innermost, most
hidden areas of our brain.

Headache disorders are notoriously difficult to classify and diagnose.
Many patients suffer from attacks whose symptoms fulfill more than one
set of explicit diagnostic criteria, and it is not infrequent that these same
attacks may change in nature with time. Is not uncommon for individuals
affected by the most severe headache disorders, such as SUNCT, cluster
headache, or hemicrania continua, to suffer from more than one type of

headache disorder at the same time. Also, especially for those who deal with recurrent headaches over a lifetime, some attacks may fulfill the criteria of completely different disorders. Less-typical attacks are not necessarily a sign of the evolution of the individual condition but just a testament to how poorly we understand this broad range of different disorders. Factors such as treatment, changes in lifestyle, aging, or just the inability to recall symptoms exactly as they were make differential diagnosis between types of headaches particularly difficult. As a matter of fact, headache disorders are among the most complicated communicable conditions to diagnose, treat, and manage in the long term.

Listing all headaches in existence clearly is beyond the purpose of this book. We will focus only on the most important ones in terms of incidence, prevalence, and significance. This chapter will focus on their characteristics, presentations, and descriptions.

EPIDEMIOLOGY AND PREVALENCE

Saying that headache is a condition that everyone has felt at some time in life is a testament to how prevalent headache disorders are worldwide. According to World Health Organization (WHO), in fact, almost half of all adults have had to suffer with one or more headache disorders at least once in any given year, and 90% of them report a history of headache across their lives. Headaches are among the most frequent symptoms seen in general practice and the most prevalent neurological disorders. They account for one-third of neurology outpatient appointments. With some small regional variations, headache disorders affect people of all races, ages, and income levels in practically every geographical area across the globe.

The most relevant headache disorders in terms of public health importance due to their prevalence and levels of disability are migraine, tension-type headache (TTH), medication-overuse headache (MOH), and cluster headache. TTH is the most prevalent one, contributing up to 60%–70% of the total headache burden. The most common headache disorders seen in headache clinics are the four subtypes of chronic daily headache (migraine, chronic TTH, new daily persistent headache, and hemicrania continua). About 1.7%–4% of the general population suffer from the most severe and disabling forms of chronic headache, which last more than 15 days per month. Chronic daily headaches are frequently associated with overuse of abortive headache medications. MOH is an iatrogenic disorder that affects more than 1% of the general population and is, by far, the most important secondary headache.

A substantial difference in prevalence between sexes has been described in migraine and other headache disorders. Depending on the headache disorder, more men than women may suffer from the condition or vice versa, with some primary headaches such as migraine showing a marked difference, with a sex ratio for lifetime prevalence of two to three females for one male. Genetic factors are likely involved in the heritability of headache disorders and underlie approximately one-third of the familial clustering of migraine. The most consistent risk factor for migraine is a family history of this condition. Headaches cause a significant cost in terms of productivity and hours of work lost since they mostly affect people in their productive years—from their late teens to their fifties. The most severe forms are associated with significant personal burden, pain, damaged quality of life, and social barriers. In the last Global Burden of Disease study, migraine alone represented the sixth-highest cause worldwide of years lost due to disability. Headache disorders collectively were second highest.

Despite their ubiquity, cost, and magnitude in pain, however, headache disorders are significantly underrecognized, underdiagnosed, and undertreated worldwide, with very few population studies fully documenting their real epidemiology. Only a minority of patients suffering from these disorders receive a professional diagnosis; about 50% of all patients resort to self-treatment without contacting any health professional. Many affected people are simply unaware that effective treatments exist. Just 40% of those with migraine or TTH and 10% of those with MOH are professionally diagnosed. On top of that, most people suffering from migraine receive neither correct diagnosis nor effective treatment. The burden of headache may very well be much higher than we are currently documenting, especially since most of the studies focus just on the highly disabling migraine rather than on the much more prevalent TTH. The average lifetime prevalence of migraine is 18% in adults and 7.7% in children and adolescents, while the lifetime prevalence of TTH is about 52%. Data from less-developed countries are even more scant, mostly due to the relatively low profile of this condition compared to communicable diseases.

PRIMARY HEADACHES

Primary headaches are those which are not the result of another medical condition. They are cyclic disorders by themselves with a complex sequence of symptoms caused by their own independent mechanisms. The *ICHD*-3 divides primary headaches into four major groups:

1. Tension-type headaches (TTHs)
2. Migraine
3. Trigeminal autonomic cephalalgias (TACs)

- Cluster headache
- Paroxysmal hemicrania
- Short-lasting unilateral neuralgiform headache attacks with conjunctival injection and tearing (SUNCT)
- Short-lasting unilateral neuralgiform headache attacks with cranial autonomic symptoms (SUNA)
- Hemicrania continua
- Trigeminal neuralgia

4.   Other primary headache disorders

These groups, however, represent a broad definition that encompasses a much more granular differentiation between individual presentations. Despite the fact that primary headaches are the most common headache type, their etiology is only vaguely understood, so they are classified according to their clinical presentation. These patterns, however, tend to vary depending on the individual affected, and they often change during a life span. Because of that, the classification criteria of primary headaches are changed and revised every so often.

Due to our poor understanding of the underlying causes of primary headaches, even this classification unavoidably misses the smaller yet probably important differences between two lifelong migraineurs. It's not infrequent for patients affected by the most severe or chronic types to switch from one headache disorder to the other over the course of their life. However, this "change" from one diagnosis to another does not necessarily reflect a true transition from one condition to a different one. Instead, it is mostly motivated by the fact that our current classifications are based on the clinical presentation of a series of multifaceted disorders that involve complicated physiological alterations of the central and autonomous nervous systems at the same time. Despite medical advances, we still fail to fully grasp the complexities of the homeostasis of the nervous system and neural functions. Knowing what really happens when they apparently stop working as they are supposed to is currently beyond our reach.

Tension-Type Headaches

TTHs are the most prevalent and common primary headaches in clinical practice. With a lifetime prevalence as high as 78%, TTHs are the most frequent headaches in the general population. They are the "normal" headache that eventually hits everyone at least once in life, with attacks that are usually self-managed and self-contained. Despite its high prevalence in the general population, the TTH is paradoxically the least studied headache disorder. The majority of research on headache has focused on migraine, so the exact causes of TTHs remain elusive even today, and treatment is based on evidence that is decades old.

The female-to-male ratio for TTHs is about five to four, but it's higher in chronic TTH (CTTH), affecting women in up to 65% of cases. Curiously enough, the prevalence of episodic TTH increases with educational level. It's hard to determine whether this population is more at risk or that more-educated patients probably seek medical attention more frequently and thereby increase the actual number of cases reported.

TTHs are also known by different names, among them, muscle contraction headaches or stress headaches. In earlier times, the diagnosis of TTH had psychological connotations (hence the name "stress headache"), as the disorder was thought to be connected with some form of mental or muscular tension. In more recent times, however, a large number of clinical and neurophysiological studies have provided convincing evidence of a neurobiological rather than psychological basis for the disorder. The pathophysiology of TTH may be different depending on the frequency of the attacks. Peripheral factors are implicated in episodic forms, whereas central factors probably underlie CCTH.

Several factors likely act as causative agents in the TTH, and the most convincing explanation is that this disorder has a multifactorial origin. In episodic TTH, myofascial pain is caused by a stimulus, usually muscle tension or psychogenic factors, that sets off trigger points in pericranial muscles. However, myofascial mechanisms have been excluded as the cause of pain; they simply represent an aggravating factor. In CCTH and more severe forms of TTH, abnormal sensitization of pain pathways in the central nervous system can be coupled with decreased ability of the body to reduce painful stimuli. Other factors, such as reduced levels of cortisol and genetic factors may be partially responsible for the abnormalities in central pain processing. Psychological stress and poor posture are other aggravating factors since they cause contraction of the neck and scalp muscles, and patients with TTH seem to have relatively weak neck-extension muscles.

Migraine

Migraines are among the most frequent primary headache disorders worldwide and are characterized by self-limited, recurrent headaches of moderate to severe intensity associated with marked autonomic symptoms. This disorder contributes to around 40%–50% of the overall headache burden, with a prevalence of approximately 14% worldwide. Alone, it accounts for 1.3% of all years of life lost to disability worldwide.

The throbbing, unilateral aspects of migraine pain are just two of the many burdens experienced by patients. This condition is, in fact, characterized by a broad range of highly disabling symptoms that include impairing nausea; vomiting; intolerance to lights, sounds, and smells; and confusion, and all of these may last for up to 72 hours. The most severe attacks are completely disabling and can significantly affect the quality of life of patients to a much more severe degree than other serious conditions such as diabetes and osteoarthritis. Some patients may have to deal with them for more than 15 days a month—literally half of their lives.

Despite having a strong genetic basis, environmental factors strongly influence how this headache disorders those who are affected. Even a simple change in lifestyle or routine can severely aggravate migraine, increasing the frequency and severity of the attacks. Trigger factors are events, changes in habits, external stimuli, or physical acts, any of which may cause or worsen an attack. They can precede an attack by as much as eight hours and are usually recurring for every individual migraineur. Some of the most common triggers include stress, coffee or other caffeinated drinks, alcoholic beverages, lack of or excess sleep, weather changes, certain foods (such as aged cheese or chocolate), food additives, and strong smells or sounds. Stress, in particular, is a trigger for nearly 70% of patients. Usually, individuals affected by migraine know their own triggers very well and do everything in their power to avoid them.

The full pathophysiology of a migraine attack is still unclear. Although several theories have tried to explain it to some extent (see the overview in chapter 3), no one of them has yet provided a fully convincing explanation of the mechanisms that generate all its symptoms. Deep stimulation of the brain eventually leads to the release of pain-producing neurotransmitters that are associated with inflammation of the head nerves and blood vessels. What brings the process to an end in the spontaneous resolution of migraine attacks is also largely uncertain.

Migraine eventually remits in 30% of subjects, generally as the patient ages over 40 or 50 or, in women, after menopause. Full remission occurs when a patient goes an entire year without migraine. In 25% of cases, however, migraine transforms into another headache disorder. Early age at onset, psychosocial stressors, high frequency of attacks, allodynia, and psychiatric comorbidity may be related to a less favorable outcome.

Trigeminal Autonomic Cephalalgias

TACs are an important subcategory of particularly disabling and painful primary headache disorders that include cluster headache, paroxysmal hemicrania, SUNCT, SUNA, and hemicrania continua. TACs are rare disorders with a genetic preponderance: patients with a family history of these conditions are at a higher risk. The most common TAC is cluster headache, with an incidence of around 0.06% to 0.1%.

All TACs are characterized by pain occurring on one side of the head with a distribution that follows the anatomical regions covered by the trigeminal nerve. These disorders also share a common presentation in terms of secondary autonomic symptoms such as eye redness, drooping eyelids, rhinorrhea (runny nose), lacrimation (secretion of tears), and miosis (contraction of the pupils). These symptoms are ipsilateral to the headache, meaning that they occur on the same side of the head where the pain is experienced. The autonomic symptomatology is partially a normal physiological response to cranial and facial pain and is found even in migraine pediatric headache disorders. However, in TACs, these symptoms are much more prominent and are associated with secondary features—such as agitation during an attack—that suggest additional sympathetic and parasympathetic dysfunctions.

Substantial differences between the four TACs are found in the duration and frequency of the attacks and in the severity of pain. The similar clinical presentation implies a common pathophysiology involving the activation of a trigeminal-parasympathetic reflex and the brain centers controlling circadian rhythms. Rhythmicity of episodes and association with sleep are central features in all TACs, which share an apparently strong bond with the human "biologic clock." Changes in everyday habits, sleep hygiene, or anything else that subverts the internal circadian and circannual rhythms—such as jet lag or transition to daylight savings time—are known triggers for TACs and can precipitate or aggravate their symptoms.

However, despite this overlap in diagnostic features, treatment seems to be extremely specific for each condition, with a marked absence of response unless medications pertaining to specific pharmacological categories are administered. Although the rather unique response to different treatments is especially helpful in establishing a differential diagnosis between the various TACs, it once again highlights our inability to frame the underlying pathophysiological mechanisms of these disorders. The distribution of pain and autonomic symptoms in TACs suggests a fundamental neurovascular implication of the trigeminal system. An inflammatory process seemingly affects both the nerves and the vascular systems immediately close to the trigeminal nerve itself, causing the release of pain-mediating neurotransmitters. Additional secondary mechanisms, such as increased intraocular pressure, endocrine alterations, and hypothalamic activation, may also be involved.

Cluster Headache

Cluster headache is a primary headache disorder characterized by excruciating pain and repeated headache episodes during the day and night. Some experts have even labeled cluster headache as one the most painful conditions known to modern medicine. You can find more information on the pain of a cluster headache in chapter 4, section "Cluster Headache." Cluster headache is also known as Horton's headache or migrainous neuralgia. (It should not be confused with Horton disease, which is a completely unrelated systemic inflammatory vasculitis also known as giant-cell arteritis, or GCA.) Patients affected by this rare type of headache that affects slightly less than one person in every 1,000 are also called "clusterheads." Although cluster headache may occur in children, age at onset is usually 20–40 years, and it's more prevalent in men than in women, with a three-to-one up to five-to-one male-to-female ratio.

Cluster headache is a highly disabling primary headache disorder characterized by circadian or circannual "clusters" or "bouts," during which the patient suffers from multiple episodes of pain (up to eight per day). These clusters may last up to several months and usually occur during the same season of the year. The pain of cluster headaches can prostrate the patients to the point they may wish to take their lives. In the past, it was also known as "suicide headache." Other secondary autonomic symptoms, such as agitation and restlessness, are also present, although it's hard to determine whether some of them may simply be caused by the unbearable intensity of the pain.

Surprisingly enough, despite the severity and dramatic nature of this syndrome, diagnosis is usually received very late, with an average interval of three to six years after onset. Between one-third and one-half of patients consult a dentist or otolaryngologist before a neurologist, probably due to the distribution of the trigeminal pain, which irradiates behind the ear and across the teeth. The presence of coexisting migrainous features and a young age at onset also contribute to delay in diagnosis.

Paroxysmal Hemicrania

Paroxysmal hemicrania is a severely debilitating primary headache disorder pertaining to the TAC subgroup. As the name implies, the hallmark of this condition is a series of frequent, unilateral (one-sided or side-locked) headaches that occur many times a day for several days in a row. Paroxysmal hemicrania is also known as Sjaastad syndrome. It is an underdiagnosed, underreported rare disease, and epidemiological studies addressing its prevalence are lacking. Paroxysmal hemicrania likely accounts for just 1%–8% of TACs and is significantly less common than cluster headache.

There are many striking similarities between cluster headache and paroxysmal hemicrania, with the latter being characterized by shorter but much more frequent attacks. However, unlike cluster headache, paroxysmal hemicrania is much more prevalent in women than in men, with a seven-to-one female-to-male prevalence. The other most obvious difference between the two conditions is that cluster headache is almost completely unresponsive to most treatments. Paroxysmal hemicrania, instead, responds completely and almost miraculously to indomethacin, an NSAID. Since the response to this drug is almost immediate and sends the condition in complete remission, it is often used to determine a differential diagnosis with other primary headache disorders.

Short-Lasting, Unilateral Neuralgiform Headache Attacks with Conjunctival Injection and Tearing (SUNCT); Short-Lasting, Unilateral Neuralgiform Headache Attacks with Cranial Autonomic Symptoms (SUNA)

Short-lasting, unilateral neuralgiform headache attacks with conjunctival injection and tearing (SUNCT) and short-lasting, unilateral neuralgiform headache attacks with cranial autonomic symptoms (SUNA) are rare primary headache disorders grouped in the TAC category. SUNCT and SUNA are characterized by sudden, extremely painful, and often spontaneous attacks lasting only a couple of seconds up to three or four minutes. They are also associated with different secondary autonomic symptoms, the presence (or absence) of which constitute the main difference between the two headache disorders.

More than 20 years ago, gender prevalence was reported with a male-to-female ratio of 7 to 1. However, back then, the condition was largely underdiagnosed and often misdiagnosed, and today, gender prevalence seems almost comparable with a male-to-female ratio of 1.3 to 1. Cases of all ages have been reported from childhood to old age, with an average onset at about 50 years. As with other TACs and migraine, familial risk is also present, suggesting a genetic predisposition toward SUNCT and SUNA. In episodic SUNCT/SUNA, attacks occur in bouts lasting from 7 days to 1 year, separated by pain-free periods lasting 1 month or more. In chronic SUNCT/SUNA, remission periods are absent or last less than 1 month. Like other TACs, bouts come during certain period of the years, suggesting a link with circadian, circannual, and seasonal rhythms. The exact pathophysiology is also unknown, although its periodicity indicates a possible relationship between the condition and the activity of the hypothalamus.

Hemicrania Continua

A particularly rare and disabling form of migraine, hemicrania continua is a dreadful primary headache that literally never stops. Albeit somewhat similar in nature and symptoms to migraine, hemicrania continua is a different and unique disorder that affects only 1.7% of total headache patients being treated in headache or neurology clinics. However, it is a highly misdiagnosed primary headache; therefore, it is largely underreported. Hemicrania continua is a chronic and persistent form of headache characterized by daily and continuous symptoms, with no pain-free periods. A diagnosis of hemicrania continua requires the headache to be strictly unilateral and go on for at least three months with no pauses between day and night. While the remitting form may leave the patient somewhat pain free for a couple of months every once in a while, the condition itself will likely stay through the entire life of the patient.

This disorder is more preponderant in women than in men, although it's still unclear to what extent. The cause and etiology of this unique disorder are almost completely unknown. Symptoms are sometimes worsened by physical exertion and alcohol use, possibly due to their effects on blood vessels. The TTH background pain usually does not hamper physical activity, causing no or very mild physical disability. The intensity of exacerbations, however, is often severe enough to resemble the worst headache disorders such as paroxysmal hemicrania or even cluster headache.

Trigeminal Neuralgia

Trigeminal neuralgia or tic douloureux is a neuropathic pain disorder caused by a disruption of the fifth cranial nerve's function. When it develops without apparent cause, it is defined as a primary disorder. When it is the result of another diagnosed condition such as a vascular dysfunction, it is defined as a secondary. The fifth cranial nerve, or trigeminal nerve, is one of the 12 pairs of nerves that are attached to the brain and one of the most widely distributed nerves in the head. It conducts sensations and pain from one side of the face, including the nose, ear, eye, and mouth, to the central nervous system.

Trigeminal neuralgia can be caused by disorders that damage the myelin sheath protecting the nerves, such as multiple sclerosis, brain lesions, or vascular abnormalities. Contact between a blood vessel or a tumor and the trigeminal nerve puts pressure on it and causes it to malfunction, leading to irritation, inflammation, and pain. Direct nerve damage such as surgical injuries, facial trauma, or stroke may also be responsible for this abnormal reaction. Trigeminal neuralgia is further subdivided in classic trigeminal neuralgia (CTN) and symptomatic trigeminal neuralgia

(STN). While the symptoms of the two forms are practically indistinguishable, STN is caused by a structural lesion, other than vascular compression, that is clinically demonstrable. CTN is, instead, an idiopathic condition occurring without any clinically evident neurological deficit. Since nerve damage can occur as a result of aging, trigeminal neuralgia is more frequently reported in people over the age of 50. The disorder has an incidence of 4.3 per 100,000 persons per year and is slightly more common in women than in men.

Other Primary Headache Disorders

In addition to the principal ones mentioned in the previous subchapters, people can experience a broad range of other, clinically heterogeneous primary headache disorders. Although these headaches can often present themselves with characteristics and features similar to secondary headaches, they're never secondary to other disorders or conditions. In other words, these disorders are never symptoms of something else, and they only share a causative relationship with physiological, nondamaging stimuli such as sleeping, ingesting cold food or beverages, coughing, or performing sexual or other physical activities. These stimuli prime a still poorly understood mechanism that leads to the generation of the headache attack and are similar to the triggers of many other primary headaches, such as migraine. However, the clinical presentation of each one of these disorders is rather unique.

Since listing the details of each one of these headaches goes beyond the purposes of this book, we will simply provide a brief description of each one of them.

- **Primary cough headache.** A brief headache that usually lasts a couple of minutes immediately after a cough stimulus. The pain is usually bilateral and posterior, reaches its peak very quickly, and then subsides. It becomes more severe when the cough is more frequent. Secondary symptoms may include vertigo, nausea, and sleep abnormalities. Cough headache is generally a secondary headache disorder associated with Arnold-Chiari malformation type I or subtentorial tumors in children. Primary cough headaches are much rarer, accounting for fewer than 1% of all headache patients consulting neurological clinics. They are usually treated with indomethacin.

- **Primary exercise headache.** A rare headache type that occurs during or after physical exercise. Pain is bilateral, pulsating, and with some features similar to migraine. It lasts from five minutes to 48 hours. It is more frequent in hot weather or at high altitude. A possible mechanism can be the incompetence of the jugular venous valve that causes

blood to flow back into the brain, causing intracranial venous congestion. Although it's usually self-limiting, indomethacin and naproxen
can be administered as preventive treatments.

- **Primary headache associated with sexual activity.** A headache precipitated by normal sexual activity that can occur before or during
orgasm. It starts as a dull, diffuse, bilateral pain during sexual arousal
that abruptly becomes more intense when climax is reached. It can
last for up to 24 hours after intercourse. It is generally more prevalent
in males than in females and can present itself for the first time at any
sexually active age. If this type of headache runs a chronic course over
more than a year, preventive treatment with indomethacin, triptans,
and propranolol can be recommended.

- **Primary thunderclap headache.** An explosive and sudden high-intensity headache of abrupt onset that can last from one hour up to 10 days.
Secondary thunderclap headache is usually associated with potentially
lethal vascular disorders such as cerebral aneurysms or reversible cerebral vasoconstriction syndrome (RCVS); therefore, it must be singled
out as a priority. The primary form is, however, benign and idiopathic.
It is associated with physical triggers such as cough, exercise, and sexual activity, but unlike the other three primary headaches, it may be
caused by any one of these triggers rather than a specific one of them.
Primary thunderclap headache is usually treated with bed rest or occasionally with vasodilator agents such as nimodipine.

- **Cold-stimulus headache.** A headache caused by exposure to a cold
stimulus applied to the head. The stimulus can be external (i.e., exposing the head to cold wind), or internal (ingestion of icy cold food or
beverages, or inhalation of freezing air). It is a common headache, frequently known as brain freeze headache or ice cream headache. Pain is
frontal or temporal, short-lasting, and usually quite intense and stabbing or piercing in nature. It is a self-limiting condition that does not
require treatment.

- **External-pressure headache.** A headache resulting from nondamaging, sustained compression of or traction upon the skin and muscles of
the head. It is different from headache attributed to head trauma, since
the compression and traction are too light to cause any significant tissue damage. It can be caused, for example, by pulling hair (traction) or
wearing a hat or tight band around the head. Pain is maximal at the side
of external pressure and can spread to nearby areas. It is a self-limiting
disorder that resolves within one hour after the stimulus is relieved.

- **Primary stabbing headache.** A headache consisting of a series of
short stabs of pain in the head lasting three seconds or less and occurring without causative agents or triggers. Primary stabbing headache

is also known as ice pick headache. The frequency of the stabbings is irregular and unpredictable, from one to many per day, and pain is usually distributed in extratrigeminal regions, unlike what occurs with migraine and TACs. In two-thirds of the patients, pain occurs in different areas of the head. Secondary, nonautonomic symptoms such as a shock-like feeling or jolting head movements can also be associated. Treatment is rarely necessary.

- **Nummular headache.** Also known as coin-shaped headache, nummular headache is characterized by small, circumscribed areas of continuous pain on the head. Pain is confined in those unchanging areas of round or elliptical shape, no larger than six centimeters in diameter (hence the name "coin-shaped"). These "coins" can be localized in any part of the scalp, although they're more frequent in the parietal region. The areas affected often show hypersensitivity to touch (allodynia), tenderness, or tactile abnormalities. Pain is chronic, continuous, and of mild to moderate intensity with occasional spontaneous or triggered exacerbations of lancinating pain that can persist for minutes or hours.

- **Hypnic headache.** A persistent headache that recurs nearly every night, waking up the patient and lasting from 15 minutes up to four hours. Attacks characteristically develop only during sleep, usually at the same time every day (hence the nickname "alarm clock" headache). Pain is TTH-like: bilateral, throbbing, and sometimes associated with migraine-like symptoms such as nausea and photophobia (sensitivity to light). Unlike cluster headache, the headache disorder most known for waking up patients at night, the pain is mild to moderate, and no autonomic symptoms or restlessness/agitation are present. Onset is after 50 years of age, and it can be treated with lithium, caffeine, melatonin, and indomethacin.

- **New daily persistent headache (NDPH).** A persistent, unremitting headache that is daily from onset, usually affecting people with no prior history of headache. The pain has no characteristic features and can mimic either migraines or TTHs, sometimes with elements of both. It can be self-limiting or refractory to treatment and can last up to several months.

SECONDARY HEADACHES

Secondary headaches can be consequences or symptoms of an underlying disease. When a new headache occurs shortly after another disorder and a direct causal relationship can be ascertained, then that headache is defined as a secondary headache attributed to the disorder. For example, when a patient develops a strong headache shortly before or after being diagnosed with a cerebral tumor, that headache is classified as a "headache caused by a tumor." This same classification remains true regardless of the characteristics of that individual headache, even if they mimic or closely resemble a primary headache disorder (such as a TTH or migraine). However, if a preexisting primary headache changes in its features, becomes chronic, or worsens in a close temporal relation to another causative disorder, then that headache is classified as both primary and secondary.

Sometimes a direct causality with another disorder can be ascertained with absolute certainty, such as in the case of orthostatic headaches that manifest while a person stands up and are relieved when the person lies down. Some other times, due to their high prevalence and frequency, headaches can occur simultaneously with another disorder by mere chance, without any direct relationship. Usually, secondary headaches cannot be distinguished from primary headache by the symptoms alone. For example, a rather unique type of headache known as thunderclap headache is characterized by a sudden, intense pain that strikes without any warning and lasts for no more than a couple of minutes. Although this headache is very often associated with potentially lethal intracranial vascular disorders, particularly subarachnoid hemorrhage and ruptured aneurysms, a benign primary form of this same disorder also exists. In general, when a direct correlation with another disorder cannot be immediately ascertained, the key lies in the features of the headache. In particular, secondary headaches can be detected when their onset is abrupt—without any warning or buildup, when the patient never experienced similar attacks in the past and describes them as "the worst one ever felt," or when the age of onset is younger than 5 years or older than 50 with no previous history of primary headache disorders.

Usually, anything that takes up space inside the head (such as a tumor or hematoma) or that affects the brain, its coverings, and the vessels of the head and neck may have headache as a symptom or consequence. In this chapter, we will mention some of the well-established causes for secondary headaches. However, in some instances, such as headache attributed to infection, the nearly endless number of possible infective causes makes it impossible to list them all. In this case, we will mention only the most relevant and well-known ones. In a few secondary headaches, the disorder may fail to remit even after the original causative agent has resolved. A typical example is a headache that was caused by a head trauma that keeps going on for years and definitely for a much longer time after the initial wound has completely healed. In this case, a secondary headache changes from the acute type to the persistent type.

Headaches Attributed to a Substance or Its Withdrawal

Headaches can be attributed to exposure to certain substances in susceptible individuals, and in some instances, can be a symptom of withdrawal from other substances. Note that this type of headache is different from a migraine, for which many of these substances represent a trigger. Many chemicals, such as nitric oxide (NO) donors and histamine, will induce an immediate headache in normal people. However, subjects affected by primary headache disorders (especially migraine, cluster headache, and TTH) may also develop a delayed headache several hours after the substance is not in their blood anymore. Similarly, susceptible individuals may suffer from this type of secondary headache even when exposed to quantities of substances such as alcohol or caffeine that are smaller than what is normally required to trigger a headache. In other words, a migraineur may suffer from alcohol-induced headaches after drinking just a few sips of beer.

Headaches attributed to a substance or its withdrawal are further subdivided into three main categories:

- Medication-overuse headaches
- Headaches caused by acute substance use or exposure
- Headaches attributed to substance withdrawal

Medication-Overuse Headaches

A MOH is a chronic daily headache caused by excessive or frequent use of headache medications (usually analgesics or pain relievers). It is the most known among the headaches attributed to a substance or its withdrawal, and the most prevalent and important secondary headache disorder. Inappropriate use of symptomatic medication for headaches for more than two or three times a week may paradoxically lead to even stronger rebound headaches.

MOHs occur as interactions between a therapeutic agent used excessively and a susceptible patient. The typical patient is usually affected by episodic primary headache disorders such as migraine and TTH, or, in some cases, cluster headache and new daily persistent headache. The mechanism through which a MOH develops depends on the drug used, and invariably, that drug was taken to stop the original headache. Lower, more frequent (daily) doses carry a greater risk than larger, less frequent (weekly) doses. Although the medications most frequently associated with MOHs are OTC analgesics and NSAIDs (due to the high accessibility of these substances to the general population), a MOH can also occur with caffeine, ergots, opioids, paracetamol, codeine, and the triptans. In particular, it happens in undiagnosed or misdiagnosed patients taking the wrong acute medication repeatedly (such as aspirin to stop migraine).

A MOH is a chronic condition that lasts for at least 15 days every month. It manifests itself as an additional headache on top of the one that was tentatively treated. Eventually, the patient starts taking the acute medication to stop both the original headache and the rebound MOH as well, in a vicious cycle that ends with the medication being taken every few hours. The pain is felt as persistent, oppressive, dull, and often present upon awakening. It can also cause a general worsening of the original headache and be present as a background pain between migraine episodes. The rebound phenomenon renders most headaches refractory to prophylactic treatment and reduces the efficacy of abortive therapy, stopping some drugs, such as the triptans, from working.

Despite being an entirely preventable and remediable disorder, MOH is one of the most common chronic and disabling diseases worldwide. With a global prevalence of 1%–2% in the general population, it represents a public health problem. MOH is probably the headache disorder causing the highest individual and social burden, with indirect loss due to reduced productivity and absenteeism accounting for about 90% of the costs. In some countries, such as Italy, Spain, and France, the individual and total national costs of MOH were estimated to be higher than for migraine. Worldwide, nearly 50% of patients with headache are primarily self-treating, and MOH is the cause of only 10% of specialist consultations. However, this disorder is very unlikely to resolve without appropriate professional care. A percentage that may fall as low as 1% in low-income countries. The absence of contact with medical professionals of this wholly avoidable disorder has a noticeable health and economic impact, representing a failure in public health care across the entire planet.

Headaches Caused by Acute Substance Use or Exposure

Headaches caused by acute substance use or exposure may occur after the exposure or ingestion of foods, medications, toxins, dangerous and nondangerous chemicals, and other substances. The causes of these headaches invariably depend on the unique mechanism of the causative agent but are often linked with a common path leading to dilation of blood vessels in the head. NO donors, such as nitrite-containing heart medicines (e.g., isosorbide mononitrate), nitroglycerin (a compound found in dynamite), or preserved meat cause strong vasodilation that may induce immediate or delayed headaches. The mechanism of headaches caused by histamine, instead, is primarily mediated via the H1 receptor and can be blocked by mepyramine.

The following substances are among those that may cause headaches in people who are exposed to them:

- Alcohol
- Cocaine
- Cannabis
- Carbon monoxide
- Certain food additives (phenylethylamine, tyramine, aspartame, and monosodium glutamate)
- NO donors (amyl nitrate, erythrityl tetranitrate, glyceryl trinitrate, isosorbide mononitrate or dinitrate, sodium nitroprusside, mannitol hexanitrate, pentaerythrityl tetranitrate)
- Histamine
- Calcitonin gene–related peptide (CGRP)
- Phosphodiesterases (PDEs)
- Acetaldehyde
- Substances containing lead (batteries, certain paints, some types of fuel)
- Substances containing benzene (turpentine, spray adhesives, inks, rubber cement, and chemical solvents)
- Headache medication (atropine, digitalis, disulfiram, hydralazine, imipramine, nicotine, nifedipine, nimodipine, sildenafil), as a common side effect occurring after occasional use
- Headache medication (combined oral contraception, hormone replacement therapy, anabolic steroids, amiodarone, lithium carbonate, nalidixic acid, thyroid hormone replacement therapy, tetracycline, and minocycline), as a direct or indirect pharmacological effect occurring after long-term use

Headaches Attributed to Substance Withdrawal

Withdrawal from headache medication and certain other substances is often associated with headache. This type of secondary headache follows and is caused by interruption of regular intake of certain substances that has lasted for at least three months. It develops in clear and close temporal relation to withdrawal of the substance. In the case of caffeine and opioids, it usually begins within 24 hours after interruption, while for estrogen withdrawal, it may take up to three days to develop. The headache will resolve spontaneously within three to seven days in the absence of further consumption. Acute headache relievers are not recommended to avoid risking development of MOH. The three principal substances known to cause headaches after withdrawal are:

- Caffeine consumed in excess of 200 milligrams per day for more than two weeks
- Opioids consumed daily for more than three months
- Exogenous estrogens consumed daily for three weeks or longer

Withdrawal from chronic use of some drugs may also cause headache. These include:

- Corticosteroids
- Tricyclic antidepressants
- Selective serotonin reuptake inhibitors (SSRIs)
- Nonsteroidal anti-inflammatory drugs (NSAIDs)

Headaches Attributed to Head or Neck Injuries

Headaches attributed to trauma or injury to the head and/or neck are secondary headache disorders that occur in close temporal relation to a structural or functional injury to the head and/or neck. They are among the most common secondary headache disorders and usually develop within one week after the traumatic event. Injuries and trauma include impact between the head and an object, penetration of the head by a foreign body, forces generated from blasts or explosions, whiplash, concussions, and the action of other external forces upon the head and/or neck. Even frequent microtraumas repeated over a long time may cause post-traumatic headaches—for example, in professional boxers or football players.

The duration varies, with most subjects recovering within days, weeks, or months. However, some people may suffer from long-term post-traumatic headache after a longer time, regardless of treatment or healing of the original injury. If the headache resolves within three months from onset, the headache is labeled as acute. If the duration extends beyond that period, the headache is, instead, persistent (previously defined as "chronic"). The persistence of the headache may also be attributed to the frequent use of abortive headache medications, which contribute to the development of medication-use headaches. Litigation and medicolegal problems are often associated with the definition of the severity and duration of headaches resulting from traumatic injury of the head and/or neck.

The pathophysiology of post-traumatic headaches is still controversial and yet to be clarified since no specific features help to distinguish them in relation to the different causative agents. Suggested mechanisms include diffuse axonal injury, neural inflammation, and/or alteration in cerebral functioning, but microscopic studies have shown subtle disruption of the nerve fibers in the brain possibly associated with the stretching or shearing forces of the trauma. A broad range of other complex mechanisms may contribute to the development of this disorder, including vascular alterations and psychogenic factors (such as the patients expecting to develop the headache).

Headaches Attributed to Cranial and/or Cervical Vascular Disorder

Several studies on animals and human subjects found robust evidence that the blood vessels of the head and neck are pain-sensitive structures that can generate powerful headaches. Many types of cranial and/or cervical vascular disorders are associated with secondary headaches that often represent a key symptom to aid their diagnosis. This correlation is so significant that in the past it was thought that the whole underlying mechanism of many primary headaches such as migraine was linked to the dilation of certain such head or neck vessels. Although we now know that the pathogenesis of such primary disorders involves several overlapping mechanisms of neurovascular origins, we still recognize that vascular disorders may cause a broad range of secondary headaches.

Although in some vascular conditions, such as ischemic stroke, headache is just one among several other symptoms, in others, such as subarachnoid hemorrhage or cerebral venous thrombosis, it is a prominent or initial warning sign. Therefore, it is important to identify this type of headache, recognize the disorder as quickly as possible, and start treatment to prevent more harmful consequences. An important clue that points to the presence of an underlying vascular condition is the sudden onset of a new, unknown headache that the patient never experienced before. Thunderclap or very abrupt headaches accompanied by focal neurological deficits are the most common phenotype of headaches caused by vascular disorders. The following list pairs headaches with the vascular conditions of which they are a secondary symptom:

- **Headache attributed to cerebral ischemic event.** A self-limiting, acute-onset headache of moderate intensity and with no specific characteristics accompanies up to one-third of cases of ischemic stroke. Headache is usually not the prominent feature of the vascular condition, and it's accompanied by focal neurological signs and/or alterations in consciousness. Albeit usually self-limiting, it is also present in a persistent form when it lasts for more than three months after the stroke has stabilized.

- **Headache attributed to nontraumatic intracerebral hemorrhage.** Headache caused by nontraumatic intracerebral hemorrhage is usually more severe than in ischemic strokes and is associated with focal neurological signs of the intracerebral bleeding itself. It is generally caused by local compression exerted by blood in the subarachnoid space. Its onset can be abrupt, and it can present as thunderclap headache.

- **Headache attributed to unruptured vascular malformation.** This headache can occur in the presence of an uncomplicated vascular malformation not associated with a hemorrhage. The vascular disorders associated with this headache include cavernous angioma, unruptured saccular aneurysms, arteriovenous malformations, dural arteriovenous fistulas, or Sturge-Weber syndrome. Depending on the type of malformation, this headache may mimic a primary headache disorder such as migraine or cluster and have an either chronic, recurrent, or self-limiting course.

- **Headache attributed to arteritis.** Headache is the most common and often sole symptom of an inflammation of central nervous system arteries (vasculitis). The presentation of this type of headache is variable, lacking specific features.

- **Headache attributed to cervical carotid or vertebral artery disorder.** Headache with or without neck or face pain is often associated with noninflammatory lesions of the cervical carotid or vertebral arteries, such as dissection. The pain is generally severe and has a sudden or thunderclap onset that is often ipsilateral to the vascular pathology. It is often recognized as an introductory symptom preceding the ischemic stroke; therefore, it should be identified as quickly as possible as a warning sign. Its presentation may sometimes be misleading and resemble migraine, cluster headache, or carotidynia.

- **Headache attributed to cerebral venous thrombosis.** Headache is a symptom of cerebral venous thrombosis (CVT) in 80%–90% of cases. It presents itself as a severe, recent-onset headache that rapidly progresses to become a persistent, throbbing pain.

- **Headache attributed to other acute intracranial vascular disorder.** Headaches can be associated with other intracranial vascular disorders and genetic vasculopathies. The list includes reversible cerebral vasoconstriction syndrome (RCVS), cerebral amyloid angiopathy (CAA), Moyamoya angiopathy (MMA), and others. Headaches can also be caused directly by certain intracranial, endarterial procedures and by cerebral angiography.

Other Secondary Headaches

There are many more headaches within and beyond the *ICHD*-3 classification. Most of them are no less relevant or painful for the people who suffer from them, yet there are simply too many for us to mention them all or provide a detailed explanation of their characteristics. However, here's a short list of some of the most important secondary headaches not included in the previous paragraphs but nonetheless worth mentioning:

- **Headache attributed to infection.** Headache is a common accompaniment of systemic viral infections such as influenza or sepsis, although it is a relatively inconspicuous symptom. It may either coexist or occur in absence of fever and may be originated by immunoinflammatory mediators together with direct effects of the microorganisms themselves. In intracranial infections such as meningitis or meningoencephalitis caused by intracranial bacteria, viruses, fungi, or other parasites, headache is usually the first and the most often present symptom.

- **Headaches attributed to psychiatric disorder.** Epidemiological data show that psychiatric disorders are often associated with headache. Headache occurs in many common psychiatric disorders, such as depression, anxiety, and post-traumatic stress disorder (PTSD). Since evidence supporting the theory that psychiatric disorders may be a direct cause of headaches is somewhat scarce, however, it has been postulated that these headaches may occur coincidentally and without causal connection. Comorbid psychiatric disorders may also worsen migraine and TTH, making them less responsive to treatment or increasing the severity and frequency of the attacks.

- **Headache attributed to temporomandibular disorder.** This headache originates in a disorder involving structures in the temporomandibular region (jaw, muscles of mastication, joints). It somewhat overlaps with TTHs, and it can be caused by muscle tension, broken bones, osteoarthritis, or degenerative diseases. It is frequently associated with diffused facial pain.

- **Headache attributed to disorder of the teeth.** Teeth disorders characterized by toothache and/or facial pain may also cause headaches. The most common causes include endodontic or periodontal infections, abscesses, traumas, or pericoronitis around a partially erupted wisdom tooth.

- **Headache attributed to disorder of the eyes, nose, or ears.** Painful disorders, lesions, or inflammations of the ears and eyes may cause headaches. Common causes include rhinosinusitis (sinus headache), conjunctivitis, acute angle-closure glaucoma, and otological pathologies.

- **Headache attributed to arterial hypertension.** An acute rise in arterial blood pressure may cause a headache but only if the increase is sudden and significant enough (e.g., to ≥180 mm Hg systolic or to ≥120 mm Hg diastolic pressure). The headache is bilateral and pulsating and remits after normalization of blood pressure. Mild or moderate chronic arterial hypertension does not cause headaches.

- **Headache attributed to hypoxia and/or hypercapnia.** Exposure to either hypoxia or hypercapnia, such as ascent to altitudes above 2,500 meters, airplane travel, sleep apnea, or diving to a depth greater than 10 meters, may cause headaches.

- **Headache attributed to intracranial neoplasia.** Anything that occupies some space inside the cranium may cause painful secondary headaches, and brain tumors are frequently responsible for this type of headache disorder. Of patients with an intracranial neoplasm, 32%–71% manifest headache as a symptom generally associated with neurological deficits, nausea and/or vomiting, and seizures.

- **Headache attributed to fasting.** Fasting for at least eight hours may cause a diffuse, mild to moderate headache in some patients, but it is relieved after eating.

- **Headache attributed to epileptic seizure.** In epileptic patients, headaches may occur within three hours after an epileptic seizure and will remit spontaneously within three days.

CONCLUSION

Headache disorders are among the most prevalent disorders of humankind. In this chapter, we examined the various types of headaches according to the current categorization, as defined by the *ICHD*-3. Although we provided a definition of the general symptoms and features of each primary and secondary headache, it should be noted that headache disorders are highly diversified and peculiar at the individual level. Each headache, and sometimes each attack, comes with its own unique features and characteristics that can change from subject to subject and, even on the same subject, over the course of lifetime. In the next chapter, we learn more about the history of headaches and how humanity learned to understand these complex disorders.

2

The History of Headaches

One half of my head [...] throbs and hammers and sizzles and bangs and swears while the other half—calm and collected—takes notes of the agonies next door.

—Rudyard Kipling

Although the diagnosis and differentiation of the various headache disorders keep evolving year after year as our understanding of them improves over time, we can be sure that headaches plagued people for as long as humanity existed. And if we have proof that some curious solution to these disorders were used by ancient societies, we can legitimately assume that prehistoric humans and hominids probably had to deal with headaches since the very beginning of humanity. We probably won't have a chance to find a pictogram of a Cro-Magnon dealing with that pesky tensive headache after a hard day's work, though.

In this chapter, we will have a brief look at the history of the first known cases of properly recognized headaches, how they were treated, and how our knowledge of this condition has evolved over the course of the last centuries. We will try to cover the most important milestones in identification, diagnosis, and treatment of headache, including treatments that didn't prove to be effective, such as drilling a hole in a patient's skull.

HEADACHE IN ANCIENT AND MEDIEVAL TIMES

In ancient times, headache was recognized both as a symptom of other diseases and as a disorder on its own. Probably the oldest observations on headaches are those dating back to the ritual texts of Mesopotamia, some 4,000 years ago. Back then, the widespread belief was that headaches were caused by evil spirits or angered gods. The Mesopotamians even acknowledged the existence of an evil spirit of headaches named Ti'u, and attributed the ailment to it. Headaches are described by several ancient Egyptian texts on medicine, such as the Hearst papyrus (2000 BCE), the Edwin Smith papyrus (1600 BCE), the Ebers Papyrus (1550 BCE), and the Brugsch papyrus (1350 BCE). Many remedies for headaches were described, even ones as strange as binding clay animal figurines to the patient's head with linen strips (probably because pressure on the head provides some temporary relief).

The first description of an ailment that was with all probability a migraine attack is found in Hippocrates of Kos's writings (460–377 BCE). He explained how the patient saw flashes darting from one eye to the other before a violent pain struck one temple, spread to the back of his head and neck, and prevented him from moving. Since vomiting provided some form of relief from the pain, he attributed migraine to vapors rising from the stomach to the head. Aretaeus of Cappadocia (30–90 CE) described unilateral headaches associated with vomiting, photophobia, sweating, and altered smell sensations. He provided the first classification of headaches by dividing them into three main types: *cephalalgia* (short, nonsevere headaches), *cephalea* (chronic headaches), and *heterocrania* (severe headaches that were likely migraines).

The first one to coin or at least use the word *migraine* is Galenus of Pergamon (129–199 CE), who described the unilateral pain of this condition as *hemicrania*, derived from the Latin *hemi* ("half") and *crania* ("skull"). He thought that the pain originated in the blood vessels inside the head and suggested a connection between the brain and the stomach due to the vomiting and nausea associated with this disorder. The word *hemicrania* kept being used across the ages, even in different cultures. It evolved from *emigranea* in Middle English and *migran* in medieval Welsh to *megrim* or *meagrim* in the early modern period. In other languages, Galenus's term still provided the common root for migraine, albeit in many variations, such as *migräne* (German), *emicrania* (Italian), *migréna* (Czech and Hungarian), *migraña* (Spanish), and *migraine* (French). Both the Greek doctor Soranus of Ephesus (98–138 CE) and Caelius Aurelianus (fl. fifth century CE) described the migraine's typical aura symptoms as fogging of vision, light flashes, and sparks resembling marble veins. Other physicians from that age, such as Pliny the Elder (23–79 CE) tried many curious treatments for severe headaches, ranging from chamomile to tying a hangman's noose around the head to placing a wreath made of fleabane on the sufferer's head.

Some doctors of the Byzantine era, such as Oribasius (320–400 CE), Aetius Amidenus (520–575 CE), and Paulus Aeginita (625–690 CE), knew and discussed headaches in their medical writings. The last one in particular described a headache associated with certain symptoms that resembled cluster headache. He also suggested that surgeons should cause immediate bleeding to save the life of patients who suffered from headaches caused by head trauma. The Islamic philosopher Avicenna (c. 980–1037 CE) explained that eating, drinking, light, and sounds could worsen the pain of migraine, and he even noted how certain smells could provoke an attack. He described migraneurs' habit of resting in a dark, silent room until the attack was over. While Avicenna suggested African ginger as a remedy to provide relief for the pain, others, such as the Arab surgeon Abulcasis, or Abu al-Qasim (936–1013 CE), resorted to more drastic approaches, such as the application of hot irons to the head of the patient, or the introduction of garlic via an incision in the temple. The first to discover a connection between headaches and hormones was Abu Bakr Mohamed Ibn Zakariya Râzi (854–925 CE), who found out that attacks would occur more frequently during menopause, after childbirth, or during dysmenorrhea.

The German nun and mystic Hildegard, Abbess of Bingen (1098–1180 CE) described a series of holy visions with vivid literary details that are now attributed to the aura of a migraine attack. She saw the appearance of a "great star most splendid and beautiful" followed by a "multitude of falling sparks" that were later turned into "black coals." During the Middle Ages, physicians such as Albert Magnus (1193–1280 CE) and Moises Maimonides (1135–1204 CE) mostly referred to the past medical writings on headaches from Hippocrates and Galen. They shared their theory that headache disorders had to be attributed to viscous humors retained in body cavities such as the stomach or brain. During that age, treatment included a broad range of mystical cures and complex herbal remedies. For example, they applied vinegar and opium poultices to the patient's head. The pores of the scalp were probably opened by the vinegar in the solution, which was allowing quick absorption of the opium through the skin.

MODERN TIMES

The introduction of the scientific method and of more empirical approaches to treatment revolutionized headache therapy in the seventeenth century. The English botanist and physician Nicholas Culpeper

(1616–1654) suggested the use of valerian to treat headaches of nervous origins in his *Pharmacopoiea Londinensis*. This remedy continued to be used into the nineteenth century and is a popular treatment to provide relief to tensive headaches caused by stress even today. The English doctor Thomas Willis (1621–1675) described three types of headaches in his medical manuals: continuous, intermittent, and intermittent with uncertain attacks. He also described many important aspects of migraine, such as the familial risk of the disease and its triggers (season changes, diet, sleep changes, etc.).

Paroxysmal hemicrania and cluster headache were first described in the first half of 1700 by, respectively, Joannes Christoph Ulricus Oppermann and Robert Whytt. Charles Darwin's grandfather, the physician Erasmus Darwin (1731–1802), was among the first to suggest that migraine could be caused by vasodilation. To provide relief from pain, he suggested that patients could be spun around in a centrifuge to force the blood to move from the head to the feet. One of the most important treatises on headaches was published in 1873 by Edward Liveing (1832–1919). His *On Megrim, Sick-Headache, and Some Allied Disorders: A Contribution to the Pathology of Nerve Storms* is a milestone in the research of migraine of headaches and is credited for proposing the mechanism of central nervous discharges (called "nerve storms") as one of the hypothetical causes of headaches and neurological conditions such as epilepsy. In 1886, the neurologist William Gowers (1845–1915) identified the higher prevalence of migraine in female patients in his medical textbook *A Manual of Diseases of the Nervous System*. He also invented a treatment for headaches known as "Gowers mixture" that contained nitroglycerin, sodium bromide, gelsemium, strychnine, nitric or hypobromic acid, and chloroform and was in use until the 1970s. In 1897, Samuel Potter's *Handbook of Materia Medica* recommended phenazone (antipyrine), cannabis, and phenacetin as valuable therapeutic agents against headaches.

Medical electricity was widely used for the treatment of migraine between the mid-eighteenth and mid-nineteenth centuries, especially after the vasomotor nerves were discovered. However, at the end of the nineteenth century, many experts criticized this approach, and new, more invasive surgical approaches were favored to remove or inhibit the activity of sympathetic nerves. In the late 1930s, Harold Wolff studied headache in the laboratory for the first time, performing several experiments to identify the vascular mechanisms of migraine. Wolff discovered that vasodilation and blood vessel abnormalities could be listed among the causes of headache disorders. Following this theory, he proposed that substances that caused vasoconstriction of dilated blood vessels could provide relief, and together with J. R. Graham, he first experimented with the effects of ergotamine. In the 1950s, following his discoveries on the vascular causes of migraine, sympatholytic surgical procedures such as vessel ligation of the carotid and middle meningeal arteries became popular strategies to treat the most severe cases of headache.

In 1941, the psychologist and migraineur Spencer Lashley published a key article on migraine aura where he proposed that visual illusions probably resulted from a phenomenon called cortical spreading depression (CSD). According to his theory, aura phenomenology such as flashes and sparks originated from a wave of excitation of the visual cortex followed by inhibition of activity. This excitation-inhibition "wave" moved at a rate of about three millimeters per minute across the brain and was later confirmed by newer brain-imaging techniques. In the early 1980s, a group of researchers in Copenhagen observed that migraine aura was associated with unique changes in local cerebral blood flow that closely matched the rate of CSD propagation.

In 2004, WHO and the nongovernmental organization Lifting The Burden launched the Global Campaign against Headache to raise awareness of headache disorders and improve the quality of headache care and access to it worldwide. In 2011, WHO published the *Atlas of Headache Disorders*, describing both the burden and the resources available to reduce headache disorders. Today, our understanding of the etiopathogenic mechanisms and causes of headache has vastly improved, especially thanks to the research undertaken by famous neurologists such as Dr. Peter Goadsby. Modern science dived much deeper in how the head and brain arteries open up during headache attacks and which neurotransmitters, such as serotonin, may be involved. New specific drugs such as the triptans have been developed to stop migraine attacks in their tracks with minimal side effects, significantly improving patients' quality of life. However, what we did understand is just the tip of the iceberg, and medical research is still a long way from fully understanding the causes of both the most severe as well as the milder forms of headache, let alone finding a final solution to treat them all in a quick and permanent fashion.

HISTORICAL NONPHARMACOLOGICAL TREATMENTS OF HEADACHE

Back when the pathophysiological mechanisms of headache were largely unknown, a broad range of treatments were tried, based on the sometimes bizarre theories that tried to explain this disorder. Before the onset of modern medicine, many curious, unique, dangerous, invasive, and often useless therapies were tried to treat the more severe and/or chronic headaches and migraines, with mixed results.

In the traditional period of humoral medicine, diseases were treated by withdrawing fluids in order to restore the right balance of the four humors (blood, phlegm, yellow bile, and black bile). After Aretaeus suggested drawing blood to reinstate *eukrasis* (humoral balance) for the first time in the second century CE, bloodletting or the application of leeches became a common practice to treat headaches. A vein or an artery in the forehead or behind an ear was incised, so it is possible that some patients found temporary relief mechanically due to the reduced blood pressure in the affected areas. Blistering was another approach suggested by Hippocrates to restore the balance of humors. The physician would apply heated glass tubes or plasters (cantharides) on the patient's skin to induce a sore and then draw blisters to "drain volatile spirits from the body." Since some of these methods required several hours of treatment (up to eight), it is possible that patients simply recovered spontaneously from migraine, as the attacks only lasted up to a certain time.

Cauterization was reserved for the most severe cases that did not respond to any other treatment. An incision was made at the patient's temples, sometimes even chiseling the bone down to the meninges, and then a red-hot iron was applied. Needless to say, this treatment caused grievous wounds from which only the most robust patients would survive. Others, such as Ali ibn Isa al-Kahhal ("the oculist"), suggested less invasive yet much more bizarre treatments, such as a dead mole applied to the patient's head. Less severe cases were treated with baths in warm, sweet waters that would help dissolve the vapors that caused the headache.

During the seventeenth century, many remedies came in the form of early modern recipe collections, such as Jane Jackson's recipe book in 1642. In her collection, Jackson described in great detail at least six different remedies to treat migraine. Most of them involved finely pounding garden worms with other substances such as fine flour, vinegar, or houseleek. The paste had to be wrapped in a linen cloth or used to made a plaster that was then bound to the patient's temples or laid on the nape of the neck. Other authors of similar recipe collections, such as Elizabeth Sleigh and Felicia Whitfield, went to great lengths to explain the usefulness of earthworms, snails, earwigs, and snakes in treating migraine. The logic behind this apparently ridiculous approach was rather simple. These creatures were "bred of putrefaction" and could be used to counteract a process of the human body that was thought to be originated from "offensive matter" that had to be expelled. These recipe books provided the basis for many of the printed medical works that proliferated in the Tudor period. Physicians of that age had no interest in experimenting with new ideas and preferred a conservative approach in order to maintain the practices of their readers and reinforce other sources of medical knowledge.

In the eighteenth and nineteenth centuries, the humoral theory was momentarily set aside, and with the advent of vasomotor theories, electricity became a new popular solution to headaches. Before electrical machines to electrocute patients were available, however, creative physicians from the Dutch Society of Sciences suggested a new type of curative bath. The patient had to hold a South American electric eel in one hand while putting the other hand on the head to find immediate relief, since the patient *"will be helped immediately, without exception."* The vasomotor theory paved the way for other nonpharmacological treatments such as arterial compression (compression of the carotid artery until the temporal pulse disappeared) and vibration therapy. The famous Georges Gilles de la Tourette, the discoverer of the homonymous syndrome, sat his patients on special vibrating chairs, because he found out that journeys in post coaches and trains could relieve the symptoms of migraine. Hydrotherapy was also popular, either through the stimulation of the feet by warm water or a hot bath with special waters or mustard. It seems that the idea of a warm bath to treat headache (with or without an eel) never fell into disuse.

The Myth of Trepanation

In addition to the earliest documented cases of headaches found in Mesopotamia and Egypt, some authors trace the history of headache treatment back to the Neolithic era. Their belief originates in the finding of some 9,000-year-old skulls that showed signs of a practice known as trepanation. This surgical procedure involved the removal of a bone segment from the skull, probably with the intent to free the evil spirits that inhabited the head of the patient and that caused the excruciating head pain. At some point in history, this procedure was certainly used for headache relief, as documented, for example, by Hippocratic texts in the fifth century BCE. Trepanation was used to reduce intracranial pressure in cases of fracture or head injury and was also identified as a remedy for such neurological or psychiatric conditions as epilepsy, madness, or paralysis. However, this type of surgery was probably used specifically and exclusively for headache relief thousands of years later than the Stone Age.

The association between trepanation and headaches may simply be a myth or unfounded speculation that originated several centuries later. During the 1870s, the French anthropologist and physician Paul Broca put his hands on a series of ancient children's skulls coming from Peru and France from the Neolithic age. Those skulls were perforated surgically—a feat that was deemed impossible by ancient civilizations that still employed simple stone tools. Since Broca was the president of the Paris Surgical Society, his discovery flared a large debate about the origins and purpose of this surgical procedure that was apparently practiced when the patient was still alive. These skulls presented no evident signs of fractures that could justify this complex surgery for mere medical reasons. Hence, it was hard to find a compelling theory that could explain the reason why a 9,000-year-old society would perform trepanation on so many youths. Broca's theory was that those people might have had special significance for ritual purposes or had "a character of sanctity." Trepanation was probably born of superstitions, to remove "confined demons" inside the head, or to create healing or fortune talismans with the bone fragments removed from the skulls of the patients. However, to provide a reason why trepanation was performed for the most part on children, he also suggested that the operation could have been performed to treat infantile conditions such as febrile seizures that would typically resolve on their own. Trepanning was not needed to treat children who experienced simple convulsions since they would have gotten better anyway. However, it may have performed due to the illusory belief that it was a necessary in order to guarantee their recovery.

The association between trepanation and headaches was established only several years later. In 1913, the world-famous American physician William Osler misinterpreted Broca's words and explained that trepanation procedures were used for mild conditions such as "infantile convulsions, headache and various cerebral diseases believed to be caused by confined demons." Osler had made Broca's theory more palatable by dropping an important fact—that these operations were performed almost exclusively on children. The idea that ancient cultures drilled holes into people's skulls to provide them relief from simple but painful conditions gained traction as the public became fascinated by it. Armchair anthropology was much in vogue, and other notorious physicians such as Sir Thomas Lauder Brunton had already tried to draw a connection between folk traditions and/or myths and common conditions such as migraine. For example, Brunton himself proposed that the zigzags of migraine aura accounted for visions of fairies and their jingling bells sound. For him and others, such as Dr. Thomas Wilson Parry, it seemed obvious that these skull holes were made by prehistorical surgeons at the request of migraineurs who wanted to expunge the demons inside their heads. Eventually, what was only unfounded speculation quickly became a fact, even if historians never collected any credible evidence to support this theory. In fact, it's highly unlikely that a child could have been treated for migraine or headache, especially because these conditions are less common in pediatric populations than in adults. However, this false belief still exists to this day even though it has been debunked already by more modern studies.

FAMOUS PEOPLE AND HISTORICAL FIGURES AFFECTED BY SEVERE HEADACHES

Migraine and other primary and secondary headache disorders make no exception when they hit; everyone, from the lowest peasant to royalty, presidents, emperors, scientists, athletes, artists, and writers may suffer from them. Many famous and influential figures of the past suffered from serious, sometimes debilitating, headache conditions that were often misunderstood. This apparently incredible high number of influential historical figures suffering from migraine led to the false belief that headaches were somehow associated with a higher intelligence or a stronger personality. In reality, it only testifies to the high prevalence and burden of these diseases and provides further evidence to how frequently they end up misdiagnosed or ignored.

These historical figures and important people were still able to change our history and have a tremendous impact on our society. While we still remember their contribution to reshape our evolution, their pain is often left out of history books and magazines. Nonetheless, their stories should empower those affected by headache disorders, as they are living proof that it is possible to leave a mark on the world even when one is affected by such a debilitating disease.

Probably one of the oldest cases of documented chronic headaches in history was Julius Caesar's, at least according to his biography, written by Plutarch. Although it was initially believed that the famous Roman general and politician was affected by migraine and epilepsy, researchers have recently debated this diagnosis and provided a new interpretation of his symptoms. Vertigo, frequent falls, sensory deficit, depression, and personality changes may, in fact, be consistent with a secondary headache caused by underlying vascular or cerebrovascular issues, such as recurrent ministrokes.

Caesar, however, was not the sole emperor who had to cope with the pain and challenges of frequent headaches. During the Han dynasty period, the Chinese emperor Tshao Tshao (Wei Thai Tsu) often required the help of the famous physician Hua Tho to treat his migraine with acupuncture. But the most popular emperor, and probably the most well-known person throughout history who was affected by severe headaches was Napoleon Bonaparte. The French conqueror suffered from attacks with increasing frequency and severity during military campaigns, but it's hard to tell whether they were migraine or, rather, TTHs originating from stress.

Early American history provides us with a brilliant example of how common migraine is and has always been. Both Robert E. Lee, the Confederate States Army general, and Ulysses S. Grant, the 18th president of the United States and the commanding Union general during the Civil War, suffered from painful and recurrent headaches. In a curious turn of events, Lee's surrender at Appomattox in 1865 was to his fellow migraineur Grant, who said that his migraines went away that same day. To lead the Union Army to victory, Grant worked closely with Abraham Lincoln. Lincoln himself also suffered from excruciating headaches that forced him to "kneel over" and be put to bed; they were later recognized as migraine.

For some people, migraine was among the drivers that later led to their important contributions to art, science, or society. For Vincent Van Gogh, migraine would represent such a tremendous burden to bear that his own frail sanity eventually crumbled under the weight and pressure of this intolerable pain. However, the illness also represented a source of inspiration that contributed to immortalizing his works. For example, it has been suggested that in the famous painting *Starry Night*, the halos around the stars were a depiction of a migraine aura. The English naturalist, geologist, and biologist Charles Darwin was plagued throughout his adult life by a number of illnesses, including recurrent, disabling headaches. His fragility, however, led to his withdrawal from society and contributed to his increase in productivity and his fruitful career in science. Despite his illness, he produced much research during his long periods of rest.

Since it's often really hard to explain migraines to someone who doesn't suffer from them, the writer Virginia Woolf used all her talent to put her personal experience on the page. Her headaches turned into a whole autobiography, and although her headaches were probably to be attributed to other underlying psychiatric disorders, she was able to describe the enormous pain of an attack and her elation and relief in its wake with incredible clarity. The German philosopher, cultural critic, poet, and scholar Friedrich Nietzsche suffered the same fate of many misdiagnosed patients affected by migraine. His psychiatric disturbances and cognitive decline have been frequently associated with a syphilitic infection. However, a more modern consultation of his biography, medical papers, letters, and other documents provided credible evidence that Nietzsche was affected by several diseases that included stroke, dementia, and migraine. In particular, the German scholar had dealt with vastly misunderstood and misdiagnosed migraine attacks since childhood.

The list of names of present and past VIPs affected by headache disorders is too long to mention them all and includes people such as Elizabeth Taylor, Thomas Jefferson, John Fitzgerald Kennedy, Sigmund Freud, Anne Frank, Elvis Presley, and many others. For better or worse, headaches affected the lives of many important people through history in the same way it affects the lives of millions of anonymous people each day.

THE INTERNATIONAL CLASSIFICATION OF HEADACHE DISORDERS

For headache disorders to be effectively managed, treated, and studied, a precise diagnosis is the first and most important step. A patient must rule out any secondary cause from which the headache may originate and that could be appropriately cured or treated. Both in clinical practice and for research purposes, separating secondary causes from primary headache disorders is crucial. A classification schema that helps identify the many different types of headaches has always been a necessary tool for making a correct diagnosis, effectively communicating the disease to the patient, and ultimately establishing proper, long-term strategies to manage the condition.

In the past, before a formal classification emerged, primary headaches were seen as a unified disease with many different presentations. More detailed advances in research contributed to the development of a new level of awareness of the existence of several discrete entities that simply shared head pain as a symptom. Eventually, headache disorders slowly obtained better recognition in clinic and nosological research, and the scientific community felt the generalized need for a universally accepted classification.

The first proposals for a consensus-oriented classification of headache disorders were the Ad Hoc Committee on Classification of Headache of the American Neurological Association (the "Ad Hoc classification") published in 1962, and a similar one from the Research Group on Migraine and Headache of the World Federation of Neurology. However, the headache disorders were simply classified into 15 types that were briefly described and with no diagnostic criteria or treatment strategies listed. The first *International Classification of Headache Disorders* was proposed in 1988 by the Headache Classification Committee of the International Headache Society (IHS), a committee consisting of more than 100 international headache experts who worked for several years on this project. The first edition of the *Classification* grouped headaches into 13 items, which were further subdivided into 165 headache types. This time, the description included clinically useful operational and diagnostic criteria and a vastly more comprehensive and hierarchical classification of headache types and subtypes.

Since the diagnostic criteria were based on the opinions of experts rather than on published and verifiable data, they were later tested on 740 subjects. The results were particularly satisfactory, with only 2 persons (0.3%) ending up having unclassifiable headache, verifying that the classification was consistent, reliable, and able to cover nearly all existing headaches. The quality of the IHS *Classification* was so high that no other classification has ever been published since then, and it was translated into more than 20 languages. The IHS classification was later revised into *The International Classification of Headache Disorders*, second edition (*ICHD-2*) in 2004, and into a third edition (*ICHD-3*) in 2018. Each update was the consequence of a better understanding of this disease and the underlying mechanisms of several subtypes, and it included newer, more granular diagnostic criteria, the recognition of additional secondary headaches, and other aspects. In the latest edition of the *ICHD*, the criteria that define each subtype of headache are based on clinical and laboratory observations and a broad range of additional studies. Today, it is universally recognized as the official classification of headaches, and it was incorporated in 1992 into the 10th edition of the *International Classification of Diseases (ICD-10)*.

CONCLUSION

In this chapter, we walked through history to know more about headaches and how we've learned to understand and manage them. We saw them through the eyes of our ancestors and explored the myths and beliefs surrounding them from the time humans walked their first steps. We also learned more about some of the most bizarre, early headache treatments while finding out how many famous historical figures have had to deal with this insidious condition. Although today we have a much better understanding of headaches as well as the help of a robust classification method to identify them, what we need to know is still more than what we know already. In the next chapter, we will discuss the potential causes of most headache disorders, how the condition is acquired, and what the risk factors are that make people more likely to acquire or manifest this condition.

3

Causes and Risk Factors

Some people spend the day in complaining of a headache,
and the night in drinking the wine that gives it.

—Johann Wolfgang von Goethe

Although virtually all people have or will experience a headache in their life, it is still unclear why some people are plagued with so many more headaches than others. Humanity has investigated the headache phenomenon for centuries, as we already saw in the previous chapter, but even science still cannot fully understand the physiopathological minutiae behind each primary and secondary headache disorder.

In this chapter, we will explore the physiological reasons why headaches occur (the pathophysiology of the condition), how this disease is acquired or inherited, and what factors (demographic, environmental, lifestyle, genetic, etc.) increase the risk for the manifestation of headaches. Since there's still no final consensus on the pathophysiology and etiopathology of most of these conditions (especially primary ones), we will present the reader with the most modern and viable hypotheses that try to explain these disorders.

AN OVERVIEW OF THE PATHOPHYSIOLOGY OF HEADACHES

Even today, our understanding of the pathophysiological mechanisms underlying primary headaches is spotty at best. While we have a general idea of how intracranial lesions or direct stimulation of internal head structures and tissue may cause most secondary headaches, we fail to fully understand what really cause migraines, trigeminal autonomic cephalalgias (TACs), and even tension headaches. Luckily enough, according to prevalence studies, headaches originate from a benign process. Though painful, primary headaches are never, in fact, inherently dangerous for the subject's physical health, and the lifetime prevalence of secondary headache resulting from threatening intracranial structural lesions is less than 2%.

Contrary to common thinking, headaches do not originate inside the brain. Since no pain receptors are present there, the brain itself is, in fact, largely insensitive to pain, at least under normal physiological conditions. To generate pain, other anatomical structures of the head and neck must be directly or indirectly stimulated through mechanical, electrical, chemical, or inflammatory action. These structures include various nerves, namely, the vagus, trigeminal, cranial, spinal, and glossopharyngeal cranial ones; the extracranial and meningeal arteries; several head and neck muscles; veins and venous sinuses; many parts of the mouth, eyes, ears, and teeth; other intracranial structures, such as the meninges, falx cerebri, and the brain stem; the skin. Thus, muscle spasms, dilation of blood vessels, infection or inflammation of the meninges, or elements that increase intracranial pressure—such as tumors—all may stimulate nociceptors.

Regardless of where it starts or which cause incited it, once it is initiated, the transmission and processing of pain are always similar. The pain receptor reacts to the stimuli by sending a message along the length of the trigeminal nerve fiber up to the brain neurons, signaling that a region of the head or neck hurts. Trigeminal fibers innervating cerebral vessels surround the large cerebral and pial vessels, large venous sinuses, and dura mater. Generally, nociceptors innervate the vessels on the same side of the trauma or stimulus, which explains the unilateral distribution of pain in certain headaches. The primary neurotransmitters and neuromodulators involved in the transmission of headache pain are glutamate, substance P, calcitonin gene–related peptide (CGRP), nitric oxide (NO), and neurokinin A.

However, we know that many primary headaches are associated with a broad range of different symptoms beyond just pain. The relative simplicity of the transmission of pain mechanism that may explain the events occurring during a secondary headache isn't even remotely enough to provide a comprehensive overview of what happens, say, during a cluster headache attack—let alone shedding a light on the complexities of a migraine aura.

Different hypotheses have been advanced over time to tentatively explain what happens in the body of the headache patient. Some of these theories hold up to a certain point and can explain at least a portion of the mechanisms behind the cascade of events that occur during a headache episode.

Pathophysiology of Migraine

The broad range of different neurological symptoms that characterize migraine suggest that multiple abnormalities in the neuronal systems influence several cortical and subcortical areas across the brain, the brain stem, and the hypothalamic and thalamic structures. The whole brain of a migraineur is probably altered at the structural, functional, and molecular levels. Studies of evoked potentials and event-related potentials have shown changes in the electrophysiology of a migraine patient brain, but how these changes should be interpreted is still a controversial matter. These abnormalities may constitute a peculiar environment that justifies the pathological mechanisms behind this disease, such as the susceptibility to changes in homeostasis and lifestyle habits, and the recurrence of headaches even when no apparent triggers are present.

In any case, the pathophysiology of migraine is complex and still not completely understood, as it certainly goes well beyond the traditional simplistic view that "migraine generator area" of the brain sends pain-producing signals to some meningeal pain receptors during a crisis. In fact, while it is probably true that migraine attacks have a central origin in those brain areas that are likely associated with aura and other neurological symptoms, nothing is known about the sequence of events that connects the prodromes (early or warning signs) with the meningeal nociceptors. That's *if* they are connected at all—something we aren't even sure about either.

Migraine prodromal symptoms suggest the involvement of several different areas of the central nervous system (CNS). Food cravings, irritability, and fatigue can be linked with abnormal hypothalamus activity; muscle tenderness and neck stiffness with the brain stem; and photophobia and hypersensitivity to sound or smell with the cortex. It's hard to tell whether these symptoms are triggered by migraine or are triggers of migraine themselves and how mechanistically different they are when they occur without headache developing (e.g., in routine circumstances).

Given the extreme susceptibility of the migraine patient to even small deviations from homeostasis (such as skipping a meal or changes in sleep habits), it can be reasonably asserted that the hypothalamic neurons regulating circadian cycles are at the origin of some of the migraine prodromes. Note that this mechanism seems to be present in TACs as well, although it is not clear to what extent. The mechanism through which a headache is initiated by the hypothalamus and brain stem is currently being explored, and several hypotheses have been suggested.

The first proposes that changes in physiological and emotional homeostasis can lead the hypothalamus into shifting the autonomic tone of the meninges toward the predominance of parasympathetic tone. This imbalance, in turn, activates meningeal receptors, causing a cascade of events that will lead to migraine pain. The second hypothesis suggests that in response to changes in physiological and emotional homeostasis, the hypothalamic and brain stem neurons can increase corticothalamic susceptibility to pain. Most nociceptive signals from the meninges are normally gated by a high brain stem tone that inhibits them. If this gating function is reduced because of a reduced brain stem tone, abnormal signals coming from trigeminovascular neurons may fire up the pain typical of the headache experience.

More in general, migraine patients may suffer from a genetic predisposition to generalized neuronal hyperexcitability. An increased activity in glutamatergic systems supposedly leads to excessive occupation of the NMDA receptor, which may have a role in amplifying and reinforcing pain transmission. The migrainous brain may be unable to manage the level of physiological or emotional stress if it becomes too high. This so-called allostatic load may not be equal at all times and depends on the sum of several external and internal conditions and on the coincidence of some of them with specific circadian phases of cyclic rhythmicity of brain stem. This could explain why the same triggers do not flare up a migraine attack at all times but only when certain (unknown) conditions are met. Similar or identical activation patterns are also found in other conditions associated with somatic pain, such as neuropathic pain, fibromyalgia, low back pain, and irritable bowel syndrome.

Eventually, the migrainous signals originating in the brain are transmitted to the trigeminovascular pathway, a plexus of nerve fibers innervating cerebral vessels that convey nociceptive information from the meninges back to the brain. Additional projections of the trigeminovascular pathway transmit neural signals to the brain stem, hypothalamic, and basal ganglia nuclei that account for some of the additional symptoms of migraine beyond just pain (e.g., loss of appetite, nausea, vomiting, lacrimation, yawning, mood disturbances, and fatigue). Cortical afferences, instead, are likely responsible for the cortically mediated symptoms typical of migraine such as allodynia, difficulty concentrating, photo and phonophobia, and amnesia, among others. Trigeminal fibers can release substance P, CGRP, and NO when the trigeminal ganglion is stimulated. These substances can generate inflammation of the dura mater and plasma extravasation, leading to migraine pain, although their action is probably not exclusive. In fact, while some drugs that inhibit neurogenic plasma extravasation, such as indomethacin, ergot alkaloids, and triptans, are egregiously effective against migraine pain, others, such as PPE blockers, substance P antagonists, and inhibitors of nitric oxide synthase (iNOS), showed no antimigraine effects in humans.

While the dura mater changes that include the sterile inflammatory response are certainly responsible for the migraine pain, it's still unclear whether they are sufficient or if other stimulators or promoters are necessary. Transient constriction and dilatation of pial arteries, mast cell degranulation, platelet aggregation, and the introduction of proinflammatory molecules, such as histamine, bradykinin, serotonin, and prostaglandins inside the meninges, are also involved.

Migraine Aura and Cortical Spreading Depression

Among the complex neurological phenomenology that accompanies migraine, the aura is probably the most iconic and misunderstood symptom. Beyond the description of its many and diversified presentations, the search for a common pathophysiological mechanism behind this symptom has been the object of many dissertations. Today, our current understanding is that a neurophysiological phenomenon known as cortical spreading depression (CSD) underlies migraine aura or is at least implicated in its generation.

CSD, or spreading depolarization, is a unique phenomenon with homogeneous characteristics that contributes to the pathogenesis of many heterogeneous clinical conditions although in a probably different way. In fact, it was first described in 1944 by Aristides A.P. Leão as a phenomenon characterizing epilepsy. Today, we know it is implicated in cerebral ischemia, hemorrhagic stroke, traumatic brain injury, and migraine aura as well, although it certainly has a different prognostic value. CSD is affected by the particular triggering event and by genetic background. While we don't know the specific processes that initiate CSD in humans, hypoxic conditions—as well as mechanisms that invoke inflammatory molecules, such as sleep deprivation or psychological stress—are known to induce it. In the most severe neurological/cerebrovascular conditions, CSD may facilitate neuronal death and further spread the physiological damage that caused it. In migraine, however, tissues are usually well-nourished tissues and otherwise healthy, so CSD is instead known to normally be a benign, self-limiting phenomenon.

CSD is a slowly propagated wave of electrophysiological hyperactivity that causes depolarization of neurons and glial cells, followed by a subsequent sustained wave of inhibition of neuronal activity due to hyperpolarization.

The hyperpolarization wave causes local suppression (depression) of the spontaneous cortical activity that spreads across the whole brain cortex as well as into other regions, such as the cerebellum, retina, and hippocampus.

CSD is accompanied by other changes at the synaptic level, the release of multiple neurotransmitters and neuromodulators, and alteration of the vascular response, blood flow, and energy metabolism. Neurons show morphological changes during CSD, including cell swelling and beading that may contribute to the release of several neurotransmitters, such as GABA and acetylcholine, in large quantities. CSD is associated with a non-linear vascular response. In damaged tissues, such as in the case of a stroke of hemorrhage, there is a widespread vasoconstrictor response. In healthy tissues, as in the case of a migraine aura, the increased electrical activity leads to the release of vasodilator factors such as NO to compensate for increased metabolic needs. Eventually, this will generate a spreading wave of vasoconstriction following the initial vasodilation, and a wave of ischemia of the cerebral tissues. Whether this ischemia is benign or not probably depends on the health of the tissues affected as well as on the events that triggered it.

We have a large body of evidence supporting the fact that CSD is the electrophysiological mechanism of migraine aura. The observation of cerebral blood flow through diagnostic imaging techniques demonstrates that migraine aura is associated with the unique pattern of changes of CSD. In particular, at the beginning of a headache attack, cerebral blood flow decreases in the posterior parts of the brain dedicated to visual perception. Then the reduced flow spreads toward the front of the brain at the same rate of CSD propagation: two to three millimeters per minute.

In any case, we still need to determine how aura may cause the actual headache or, at least, how these two symptoms are linked. A drastic depolarization is known to release a broad range of noxious substances including proinflammatory molecules and ions, CGRP, substance P, and NO. It has been suggested that depolarization occurring during CSD causes these substances to be released and then introduced into the meninges. Here they stimulate the nociceptors of the trigeminovascular system and trigger the headache.

Substances associated with improvements in ion channel function, such as acetazolamide, lamotrigine, and other antiepileptic drugs, have been shown to decrease the frequency of attacks. The prevention of migraine aura possibly occurs due to the suppression of CSD, although it's unclear why these drugs are also effective in preventing headaches even in patients suffering from migraine without aura. The actual link between SD and migraine without aura is, in fact, poorly understood. It has been speculated that CSD may either affect silent subcortical regions or fail to reach a clinically detectable threshold.

Pathophysiology of TACs

The current classification of TACs identifies a series of somewhat different headache disorders that are grouped together because of a similar clinical presentation and a suspected common pathophysiological mechanism. In particular, this common underlying mechanism apparently involves the trigeminovascular system, the trigemino-parasympathetic reflex, and centers controlling circadian rhythms. Any pathophysiological model that tries to describe TACs must account for their three major characteristics: trigeminal pain, autonomic signs, and the distinct circadian rhythmicity, particularly in cluster headache.

Currently, no consensus has been reached on whether the pain has a central rather than peripheral origin. However, a purely peripheral model fails to provide a convincing explanation for several features of primary TACs, such as the selective gender prevalence, association with sleep patterns and circadian rhythms, and the often strictly unilaterality of the symptoms. Positron emission tomography (PET) and other diagnostic imaging techniques have identified the posterior hypothalamus as a key region in the central generation and termination of TAC headache attacks. The posterolateral region of the hypothalamus in particular is the area more highly associated with cluster headache since it regulates the sleep-wake cycle. An alteration in the production of some hypothalamic neurotransmitters such as melatonin may also account for the peculiarly cyclic patterns of cluster headache across the day and across the year (seasonality).

The distribution of pain in TACs is explained with the implication of the trigeminovascular system, which is hypothetically involved after hypothalamic activation together with the cranial autonomic system. However, hypothalamic peptides Orexin A and B can both induce or suppress pain in the trigeminovascular system, showing how dysfunctions in this brain area likely have a more complex role in the whole pathophysiology mechanism of TACs. Currently, the interrelations of hypothalamic regions with the trigeminal autonomic reflex are yet to be determined. Also, it's still unclear whether these hypothalamic alterations are part of the etiology of TACs or are the consequence of certain pain conditions in general.

Notably enough, the trigeminovascular system is the same pathway implicated in other primary conditions, such as migraine. Together with some of the hypothalamic alterations, its activation has been detected in other primary headache conditions, including hemicrania continua as well as migraine. Although this shows how the pathways involved in TACs are somehow akin to the ones involved in migraine, especially when overlapping is present in comorbid patients, some fundamental differences between the primary headache disorders must be noted. For example, unlike in less severe migraine attacks, CGRP levels in cluster headache and chronic paroxysmal hemicrania are particularly elevated. In addition, the much higher degree of cranial autonomic activation does not just account for a much more significant pain suffered by the patient but can also explain the difference between TACs and migraine in relation to autonomic manifestations. Since many cluster headache patients suffer from pain outside the trigeminal dermatomes, it is possible that their uniquely unbearable pain may have a different central origin beyond the trigeminal system.

Sympathetic symptoms such as miosis and ptosis (drooping or sagging) may be linked with a generalized sympathetic dysfunction, at least in paroxysmal hemicrania. Since in cluster headache, autonomic symptoms can occur without pain or be absent altogether, this sympathetic dysfunction is not, however, a driving force. In SUNCT and paroxysmal hemicrania, neuropathic mechanisms may be involved, since in both these conditions, attacks can be triggered by mechanical stimulation. Perivascular neurogenic inflammatory processes can worsen symptoms or increase pain in cluster headache and paroxysmal hemicrania. Dilated blood vessels may contribute in stimulating trigeminal nociceptors directly, although they cannot be the origin of pain, since even suppression of vasodilation does not stop it once it's started.

Pathophysiology of Tension-Type Headache (TTH)

The pathophysiology and pathogenetic mechanisms of TTH remain largely unclear. Several theories have been suggested, but while muscular and psychogenic factors are believed to be central in the genesis of TTH, the complete pathophysiology is likely multifactorial in nature. The original theory was that prolonged muscular contraction due to a wrong posture, anatomic abnormalities leading to cervical instability, or psychogenic stress would eventually lead to the release of pain-mediating substances. The muscular origin of the pain has been determined by recognizing the presentation of the pain, which tends to be achy, dull, poorly localized, and radiating. Myofascial pain occurs once a trigger point in pericranial muscles is stimulated, although myofascial mechanisms on their own simply represent an aggravating factor. Electromyograms (EMGs), in fact, often fail to detect the supposed increased resting-muscle tension that should correspond with the headache pain. It has been speculated that in patients with chronic TTH, muscle hardness can be permanently altered, leading to abnormal nociceptive stimuli. NO is also known to be a local mediator of pain in the affected areas.

Conversion of episodic to chronic TTH probably occurs due to prolonged nociceptive input from peripheral pericranial myofascial tissues.

Hypersensitization of supraspinal neurons will eventually decrease the pain threshold in cephalic regions up to a point where even simple palpation or pressure in the head and neck will cause pain. On top of that, the body may reduce its ability to stop painful stimuli to the supraspinal structures because of decreased antinociception. Cortisol levels can be reduced in patients suffering from chronic tension headaches for longer than five years. Cortisol is a potent anti-inflammatory substance that modulates inflammation and stress response. It is possible that reduced cortisol levels are caused by hippocampus atrophy resulting from chronic stress. In the end, the continued and prolonged stimulation of the central nervous system will cause it to misinterpret innocuous stimuli as painful ones, inducing and maintaining a chronic sensation of pain in the temporal region. In any case, abnormal or increased sensitivity to pericranial myofascial pain may be central in patients with TTH.

Etiopathology of Trigeminal Neuralgia

Currently, there are several popular theories that try to explain the etiopathology of trigeminal neuralgia. A polyetiologic origin of this condition has been suggested, since in patients suffering from trigeminal neuralgia, comorbidity with vascular diseases such as atherosclerosis and arterial hypertonia, and multiple sclerosis, allergies, and diabetes has been frequently reported. However, there is no evidence supporting a direct relationship between trigeminal neuralgia and other neurologic, vascular, neurodegenerative, or autoimmune disorders. In fact, for the majority of patients, there is no identifiable cause.

Trigeminal neuralgia may be associated with morphological and functional disturbances of the trigeminal nerve system's vasculature, which can have influence on the pathogenesis of the disease. However, numerous autoptic studies show that many patients didn't suffer from trigeminal neuralgia even when clear morphological changes in blood vessels were noted. Up to 15% of patients diagnosed with this disorder develop multiple sclerosis. On the other hand, no more than 4.5% of patients with multiple sclerosis develop trigeminal neuralgia. This may suggest that, in those suffering from both these disorders, trigeminal neuralgia may be just a symptom of multiple sclerosis itself rather than being caused by it.

Diabetes mellitus can be a causative factor for trigeminal neuralgia since it frequently affects the trigeminal nerve function, even if in most cases this occurs in a subclinical fashion. Otolaryngological pathologies such as sinusitis, periostitis, periodontitis, and dental cysts are frequently reported, with some authors stating that nearly 90% of patients had history of inflammatory disorders of the ear, nose, and throat region. A popular etiologic theory is that a neurovascular compression at the root entry zone can lead to demyelination and a dysregulation of neural transmission. Reasons for neurovascular compression include arteriovenous malformations, tuberculomas, cysts, and tumors that may directly compress the nerve root or cause its displacement through distortion of the contents of the posterior fossa. However, many patients with trigeminal neuralgia have no identifiable mass that may cause compression, and even if they have, neuralgia may occur on the opposite side of the mass lesion. Lastly, neurovascular compression is also observed in asymptomatic patients.

The allergic hypothesis has been proposed to account for the higher levels of histamine in the blood of trigeminal neuralgia patients. Clinical symptoms can be rapidly precipitated by provocative endogenous and exogenous factors that can trigger local immune response (such as getting cold, rhinitis, seasonal allergies, etc.). Histamine release probably plays an important role in the pathogenesis of this condition, but there's still no direct evidence supporting the idea that allergies are the primary causative agent for trigeminal neuralgia.

Pathogenesis of trigeminal neuralgia is also largely unclear, and there's a distinct lack of objective evidence to support any of the controversial theories that try to explain this disorder. Together with the absence of a univocal etiologic agent, the highly dynamic nature of trigeminal neuralgia pain makes it difficult to explain the disorder in purely anatomical terms. A progressive dystrophy in the peripheral branches of the trigeminal nerve is observed, with local changes including demyelination at the entry zone of the trigeminal nerve and atrophy or hypertrophy of peripheral axons. Whether these structural changes are caused by neurovascular compression or allergic-immune reactions, the final effect is a pathologic state of paroxysmal irritation leading to ectopic neural activity. Aberrant impulses are fired across damaged nerve fibers that cannot contain them anymore, leading to sudden bursts of unmitigated pain. Disorders that cause local vascular, immune, or neurological alterations such as atherosclerosis, multiple sclerosis, diabetes, chronic allergies, and neuropathic pain can further weaken the neurohumoral barrier complex and its compensatory mechanisms. They can either represent an etiologic factor or simply a more favorable condition to the development of the pathogenetic mechanism of trigeminal neuralgia.

RISK FACTORS AND TRIGGERS

Albeit very few people never experience a single headache in their lifetime, primary headache disorders are associated with several physiological, genetic, lifestyle, environmental, and psychological risk factors. In addition, some primary headaches, such as migraine, cluster headache, and paroxysmal hemicrania may flare up from a broad range of different triggers. More than three-quarters of migraineurs are, in fact, able to identify at least one trigger for their headaches, usually environmental causes such as weather, stress, or certain food. These triggers obviously go beyond those factors generating secondary headaches such as drug assumption in medication-overuse headache (MOH) or alcohol consumption in hangover headache.

Most risk factors are associated with illness chronicity (chronicization) or general worsening of the condition (e.g., attacks last longer, are more painful, and occur more frequently). The rest of this section is devoted to particular risk factors.

Gender

Certain headache disorders affect the two genders disproportionately. For example, men are more likely to have cluster headaches than women, with a prevalence of three to one up to five to one. Migraine prevalence, on the other hand, disproportionately affects women since it's present in approximately 18% of females versus 6% of males in the United States. Migraine in particular may be linked to specific hormone fluctuations, such as those seen just prior to menstruation (which is a trigger for this condition on its own). In fact, more than half (55%) of women suffer from menstrual migraine, and the majority of them show improvement in frequency and/or severity with menopause or pregnancy.

Age

For both migraine and TTH, the highest prevalence occurs between ages 35 and 39 years, although prevalence is still high in the group aged 15–49 years. Puberty is the time when migraine starts becoming more prevalent in women than in men. For other headaches, such as chronic daily headache, prevalence appears to be fairly constant throughout adulthood.

Socioeconomic Status

The relation between headache and socioeconomic status (SES) is still controversial. While some studies point a direct relation between lower SES and headache-disorder incidence, prevalence, and a poorer prognosis, others seem to differ. Previously, it was postulated that headache was mainly a disorder of high-income countries and particularly prevalent among the wealthier populations. Today, this notion has been refuted, at least in part, since no clear patterns between prevalence of migraine or TTH and SES can be drawn. However, while this link is probably impossible to determine on a global scale, it may be true that socioeconomic development factors may have a critical importance as risk factors in some countries or regions.

Psychological Stressors

Stress seems to be a trigger and a risk factor for nearly all types of primary headache. Social and psychological circumstances that challenge the adaptive capabilities of an organism can have a negative impact on patients affected by headache disorders. A broad range of common headache triggers may be associated with a stressful life as well, such as sleep disturbances, changes in sleep patterns, fatigue, skipping meals or not eating in time, anxiety, and/or depression. Stressful life events such as death of loved ones, changes in marital status, parental separation, job loss, and relocations may have a precipitating effect. Negative life events in particular can have the highest negative impact on the condition as a whole when compared with any other risk factor. People who experienced the most negative life events are those who report a higher frequency of migraine symptoms and a longer history of migraine symptoms, and they are more likely to experience comorbid disorders.

Occupational factors may also play a significant role, especially for those professionals who must deal with heavy workloads on a regular basis and experience states of high tension and high intensity for long periods. Comorbidity with a psychiatric condition is a risk factor on its own for transformation of migraine into a chronic form or for development of medication-overuse headache.

Environmental Factors

Weather or climate changes may lead to imbalances in homeostasis, requiring adjustment and adaptation that may trigger or precipitate headaches. Many environmental changes, such as changes in humidity, temperature (too hot or too cold), and barometric pressure, as well as strong winds and storms, can act as triggers for migraine, TACs, and TTH. Many patients affected by migraine are sensitive to motion sickness as well, so deep-sea diving, flying in airplanes, and traveling by car, train, or boat can also have the same effect. Bright or flickering lights, glare, and light reflections on water, sand, snow or through clouds, as well as loud sounds and noises, can have an irritating effect on sensitive patients.

Lifestyle Factors

Exposure to certain foods or chemicals is known to increase the frequency or severity of headache attacks and likely act as a trigger. Vaporized substances such as carbon monoxide, nitrites, and fumes from faulty furnaces can reduce blood oxygen levels and cause vascular changes that are known to worsen migraine and cluster headache. Because of this, smoking (both active and passive) is often a risk factor. Similarly, alcohol consumption as well as certain dietary habits represents both risk factors and triggers, especially when the patient consumes foods containing glutamate, nitrites, caffeine, or tyramine in high amounts. Obesity and a high body mass index (BMI) are also predictive of higher incidence and prevalence of many headache disorders.

Physical and Physiological Factors

Comorbidity with other chronic pain syndromes (such as arthritis and musculoskeletal pain) may increase the risk for co-occurrence of certain types of headaches, especially chronic ones. Lifetime injuries to the head or neck are also associated with an increased risk of headache, but discrepant results exist due to differences in severity or type of injury and latency between injury and development of headache (which may very well be secondary rather than primary). Some types of acute facial or head pain, such as toothache or otitis, as well as overexertion (straining, lifting, bending) may act as triggers for migraine or TTH, or, in contrast, act as abortive measures to stop cluster headache attacks. Stimuli affecting the olfactory nerves, such as strong odors and perfumes, or conditions such as sinus infections or allergies may trigger migraine and cluster headache. Lastly, some apparently harmless physical stimuli such as chewing, brushing teeth, or shaving may trigger SUNCT/SUNA and trigeminal neuralgia.

Familial Risk and Genetics

Familial risk for headache is a strong predictive factor for some primary headache disorder. Headaches tend to run in families, especially migraine. Nearly 90% of patients have a family history of migraine, and the risk of suffering from this condition is up to 75% if at least one parent suffers from it. For other headaches, an increased familial risk suggests that genetics are likely involved, though the extent to which familial risk with a primary headache disorder represents a risk factor.

GENETIC CAUSES AND BIOMARKERS

Primary headaches are multifactorial disorders, likely caused by a mix of genetic and environmental factors, the patients' unique life histories, and their individual lifestyle choices. All these factors may account for the observed clinical heterogeneity of most primary headaches, although it's still clear we're missing many pieces of this incredibly complex jigsaw.

A genetic predisposition to migraine was first observed in patients with familial hemiplegic migraine. Large genome-wide association studies have identified a total of 13 susceptibility gene variants for migraine with and without aura. Candidate genes include neurological, vascular, inflammatory, and even hormonal genes. Modifications in genes related with estrogen and progesterone metabolism may account for the different gender prevalence of this disease and the association with menstrual migraine. The search for biomarkers of migraine unexpectedly proved to be instrumental in shedding a light on the still obscure pathogenetic mechanisms of this condition. Rather than just confirming the diagnosis, the identification of specific genes helped researchers establish a vector toward the current neuronal hyperexcitability hypothesis. Alterations have been found in the genes that regulate glutamate availability in the synapses, and in other genes that regulate synaptic development and plasticity. Although we can't confirm our current speculations, it is reasonably to infer that a migraineur's brain isn't properly wired to set a normal level of habituation. Other than providing a convincing explanation of the multifactorial nature of this primary headache, these genetic findings may indicate that the structural alterations found in the brain of a migraine patients are inherited and not caused by the condition.

Unlike in migraine, gene discoveries in other types of headaches are essentially lacking. For cluster headache, even if the genetics are still unclear, a certain degree of familial risk has been observed, especially in first-degree relatives who have a 14-fold increased risk. However, the pattern of inheritance does not appear to be uniform. Both autosomal recessive and dominant genes with low penetrance can be involved, but a multifactorial inheritance may also be possible. In particular, a significant association was found with a hypocretin receptor 2 (HCRTR2) gene polymorphism, but more evidence is needed. Polymorphism in some genes may account for the different treatment response to triptans that causes roughly 30% of cluster headache patients to find these medications ineffective. Familial SUNCT occurring in siblings has also been reported, raising the possibility that a genetic predisposition may be behind other TACs as well.

For TTH, the situation is a bit more complicated. Infrequent episodic TTH seems to be caused primarily by environmental factors. In frequent episodic and chronic TTH, genetic factors may also have a role, but only a few molecular genetic studies have been performed.

CONCLUSION

Once a trigger fires up an attack, patients affected by a primary headache disorder know they're headed for a world of pain. Knowing these triggers as well as the risk factors of most primary headaches is paramount to prevent, reduce, or at least be prepared for such attacks. In this chapter we discussed them together with pathophysiological mechanisms that generate and maintain the pain and secondary symptoms of the major headache disorders we know. We also explored the possible genetic causes behind them, and the biomarkers used to identify the genetic changes occurring in patients affected.

In the next chapter, we will focus on the most empiric aspects of headaches: how they present themselves and what their signs and symptoms are. This is important to identify each individual headache disorder, to manage it, and to guarantee the most acceptable quality of life to each patient.

4

Signs and Symptoms

And then a throb hits you on the left side of the head so hard that your head bobs to the right. ... There's no way that came from inside your head, you think. That's no metaphysical crisis. God just punched you in the face.

—Andrew Levy

The symptoms of a condition are the aspects that a patient may notice, while the signs are the features of a disorder that a doctor may notice upon examination. Signs, in particular, are used to ease the differential diagnosis, which, in this case, is a particularly delicate issue since the borders that define many headache disorders frequently tend to overlap.

When it comes to headaches, determining signs and symptoms with enough accuracy is an arduous feat. Assessing the severity and impact of headaches is hard, especially given the enormous differences between the clinical presentation of the various types of headache disorders. The symptoms of a migraine are very different from those of a tension-type headache (TTH) and may also show that the very nature and origin of these two conditions can be completely different. It may be an exaggeration, but it's nonetheless true, to some extent, that the only characteristic in common among the various headache disorders is that the pain originates in the anatomical region of the head. On top of that, even when a patient suffers from a headache that can be traced back to a specific diagnosis (e.g., a cluster headache rather than a paroxysmal hemicrania), ultimately that patient's clinical presentation may be very different in comparison to that of another patient.

Individual characteristics as well as many unknown factors likely affect the intensity, frequency, severity, and features of a given headache disorder's symptoms. It is not infrequent that the clinical features of an individual headache may also change at its onset and as the condition progresses or evolves. Therefore, the descriptions included in this chapter should not be taken as absolute, especially for those headache disorders that are inherently characterized by a broad diversity in clinical presentation (one example above all: migraines). Since there are many different types of headaches, this chapter will take a brief overview of the most characteristics signs and symptoms of some of the principal types.

TENSION-TYPE HEADACHE (TTH)

TTH are broadly categorized into infrequent episodic TTH (less than one episode of headache per month); frequent episodic TTH (between 2 and 14 episodes of headache per month for at least three months every year); and chronic TTH (more than 180 days per year). It should be noted, however, that infrequent episodic TTHs are rarely diagnosed, since patients seek medical help only in rare instances. Less frequent attacks are usually self-treated with over-the-counter (OTC) analgesics and nonsteroidal anti-inflammatory drugs (NSAIDs) without specific need for medical attention. A definition of probable TTH is also included in the *ICHD*-3. It encompasses all those cases that are hard to distinguish from early-phase migraines since the diagnosis of this type of headache disorder essentially relies only on symptoms.

Chronic TTH (CTTH) is a more serious and highly disabling disorder that often evolves from episodic tension-type headache and usually requires medical consultation. It affects 2%–4% of the population, and generally lasts for the greater part of a lifetime. However, even patients affected by CTTH frequently delay consultation until disability and frequency become so high as to be unbearable. In one study, two-thirds of patients who suffered from daily or nearly daily TTH episodes waited for an average of seven years before seeking medical attention.

The pain of TTH is usually described by patient as a dull bilateral sensation of pressure and constriction in the temples and back of the head. This sensation is often described as "wearing a tight band around the head" or like a heavy burden on the head. The intensity is mild to moderate and is often associated with muscle tightness. An episode may last from

30 minutes to up to a full week, with pain usually increasing slowly throughout the day until it reaches a plateau. Unlike migraine, it's not aggravated by physical exercises and routine activity, and it is bilateral in 90% of the cases. Pain can also be felt behind or inside the head as well. TTH pain is usually not associated with other neurological or autonomic symptoms, except for photophobia or phonophobia, which are, however, mutually exclusive. Psychological tension, lack of sleep, alcohol, menstruation, and not eating are all both common TTH triggers and headache-aggravating factors at the same time.

MIGRAINE

Migraine attacks are usually preceded by a series of premonitory symptoms that occur a few hours before onset of pain. This prodrome phase is characterized by a broad range of different phenomena ranging from altered mood, fatigue, muscular rigidity, craving for certain foods, and motor or vision disturbances. Prodromal symptoms are associated with hyperactivity of the limbic system and hypothalamus. In roughly 25% of migraine sufferers, these visual effects (defined as "aura") are particularly pronounced and may last for up to 60 minutes. See the following subsection for more information about migraine aura. After a migraine attack is over, the patient may feel confused and exhausted—suffering from impaired thinking and blurry vision—or euphoric and refreshed for several hours. This phase is called "postdrome" and may vary each time in some individuals.

Migraine pain is usually localized on one side of the head, generally on the temple, behind the ear, and/or around the eye and nose. It is pulsating in form, and it's usually aggravated by routine physical activity. Runny nose, tight jaw, and watery, reddened eyes are also frequent, as well as pain reaching the teeth, as the trigeminal nerve is involved. The pain may occur (1) on the left or right side of the head, (2) always on the same side, or (3) even on both sides at once. Some patients experience different types of migraine attack depending on the side of the head—such as the stronger ones always hitting a preferred side.

Pain in the head is just the tip of the iceberg, and it is usually not the most disabling symptom for a patient affected by migraine. Strong nausea, vomit, lack of balance, a generalized feeling of malaise, confusion, loss of vision, and hypersensitivity or intolerance to sounds, lights, or smells all characterize this condition, which is often severely disabling—well beyond a simple headache. An attack usually lasts between 4 and 12 hours but may last for up to two or three days. A migraine lasting longer than 72 hours is classified as *status migrainosus*.

The severity of an attack may range from mildly tolerable to completely disabling. The severity of the condition itself is also highly variable. One-quarter of migraineurs experience more than four severe attacks per month, nearly half have between one and four severe attacks, and 38% have less than one severe attack per month. When migraine hits more than 15 days a month, it is classified as chronic. Migraineurs are typically depicted as heavily prostrated individuals forced to crawl in fetal position into a dark corner as they endure never-ending suffering. Depending on the severity and length of the attack, the patient may be completely unable to perform any activity for hours or even days. Given its frequent comorbidity with disorders such as anxiety, depression, allergies, and chronic pain disorders, migraine reduces the quality of life of those affected more than diabetes or osteoarthritis do.

Migraine is also frequently associated with allodynia, a form of pain hypersensitivity associated with nonpainful stimulation. A subject affected by allodynia may become so sensitive to touch during a migraine attack that even a light touch or mild change in temperature may produce pain and discomfort. Allodynia in migraine results from inflammation of the nerves surrounding the blood vessels on the brain surface. Repeated and prolonged central sensitization of these nerves during an attack causes them to become hyperexcitable, transforming normal signals such as touch on the scalp and face into abnormal painful responses.

Migraine Aura

The migraine aura is a series of sensory disturbances and hallucinations that occur during the prodromal phase of the migraine, shortly before an attack. Often described as a "warning sign," aura affects only 25%–30% of migraineurs, and it generally doesn't occur during every headache episode. In some instances, the aura is neither accompanied nor followed by headache of any sort.

Symptoms of aura include vision, sensory, and motor disturbances, with visual aura being the most common type, occurring in over 90% of patients. Motor disturbances are the least frequent symptoms. Disturbances include flashes or sparks of light, bright dots or zigzag lines that float across the field of vision, blind spots (scotoma), tingling or numbness on one side of the face or body, vertigo, inability to speak clearly, motor impairment, and muscle weakness. They usually last 20–60 minutes. Patients experiencing sensory or motor symptoms in the extremities and/or speech or language impairment almost always also experience visual aura symptoms during the attack. Multiple symptoms usually follow one another in a defined succession: first the visual, then the sensory, and finally the aphasic.

A relatively small number of patients (less than 10%) suffer from rarer forms of migraine with aura. These are classified as separated subtypes because of genetic and pathophysiological differences from typical aura. The rare forms of migraine with aura are:

- **Migraine with brain stem aura.** A migraine with aura symptoms arising from the base of the brain (brain stem) and without motor symptoms. Brain steam aura symptoms include slurred speech, vertigo, tinnitus, double vision, uncoordinated movements (ataxia), and impaired hearing. Brain stem aura may occasionally happen to anyone who experiences migraine with aura.

- **Hemiplegic migraine.** An aura that includes transient motor weakness or paralysis on one side of the body (hemiplegia). Additional symptoms can range from ataxia, fever, and confusion up to profound coma. The weakness will resolve completely, and it typically goes away within 24 hours, but it may last for several days.

- **Retinal migraine.** An aura with visual disturbances occurring in one eye only. Patient can only experience them while looking through the affected eye, which may also become temporarily blind. Monocular disturbances are always fully reversible.

The causes and mechanisms of migraine with aura aren't entirely understood. Evidence shows that, before or simultaneously with the onset of aura symptoms, an electrical or chemical wave of nerve cell activity spreads across the brain and excites the trigeminal nerve and the visual cortex. This phenomenon is known as cortical spreading depression (CSD) and is characterized by a local and transient reduction of cerebral blood flow that causes a suppression of spontaneous electrical activity in the brain. This depression moves slowly as a wave, starting posteriorly and then spreading anteriorly. After some hours, blood gradually flows back, causing vasodilation, hyperemia, hyperexcitation, and an inflammatory process that can ultimately lead to the genesis of migraine attacks and aura symptoms.

Other than causing sensory disturbances, the migraine aura doesn't affect the pathophysiological features of the disorder (i.e., duration of the attack, frequency, intensity, response to treatment, triggers, etc.). Migraine with aura is treated and prevented with the same medications and self-care measures (sleep hygiene, dietary habits) used for migraine without aura. Triptans and ergotamines are currently contraindicated in the treatment of hemiplegic migraine and brain stem aura because of their vasoconstrictive properties and possible safety issues associated with a risk of vessel spasm and stroke.

CLUSTER HEADACHE

A unique feature of cluster headache is the distinctive circadian and circannual periodicity of the attacks, which occur during specific active periods called "clusters" or "bouts." During a cluster, the patient will suffer from one to four (sometimes up to eight) attacks per day, whose duration ranges from 30–90 minutes. The pain reaches its most agonizing peak after 5 or 10 minutes and then stops quite abruptly when the episode is over. Headaches strike during certain specific times of the day or night, often at a set time and frequently waking up the subjects one or two hours after they have gone to sleep. During a cluster, the patient is especially vulnerable to certain triggers that induce extra attacks within a few minutes, including the ingestion of alcohol, strong smells such as perfumes or paints, hunger, or strong emotions. In contrast to migraine, intense physical activity may abort or temporarily ameliorate an ongoing attack.

Cluster headache bouts usually last for one to three months, with seasonal active periods occurring during the same season each year (i.e., from January to March). Correlation between changes in daylight hours or seasonal changes is quite frequent. Curiously enough, the whole cluster seems to mimic the individual episodes on a macroscopic level. Long-term patients report shorter and less severe attacks during the onset phase of each cluster period until a plateau is reached, and bouts often end up quite abruptly as well. When the cluster period is over, patients remain pain free during remission periods of months or years. If this remission period lasts for at least one month, the patient suffers from episodic cluster headache (ECH). People who do not have a remission period of at least a month between clusters that last for at least one year are a minority (10%–20%) and suffer from chronic cluster headache (CCH). Patients may transition back and forth from ECH to CCH, suggesting a common mechanism behind both forms of this disorder.

The pain is strictly unilateral, piercing, stabbing, throbbing, or burning in nature and usually follows the traditional distribution of other trigeminal autonomic cephalalgias (TACs), so it is centered around eye, temple, and forehead region. Due to its high intensity, nerve overstimulation and diffused inflammation may cause it to spread to nearby areas as well, making the diagnosis more complicated since it's based on the clinical presentation. Cluster headache episodes are marked by distinct autonomic symptoms, namely conjunctival injection, rhinorrhea (runny nose), nasal congestion, forehead and facial sweating, miosis, and ptosis. Most patients are characteristically agitated and restless for the whole duration of the attacks. The secondary autonomic symptoms are more marked in cluster headache than in other TACs. Note that due to the severity of the pain, other symptoms such as nausea or vomiting may also be present, but, unlike migraine, they are more a reaction to the intensity of the stimulation and stress rather than primary features.

The Unbearable Pain of a Cluster Headache

Routinely reaching the maximum level of the most well-recognized severity scales, the pain of a cluster headache can be hardly described with simple words. Every patient usually comes up with a unique description of a sensation that is so intense that it has its own unique way to bore through the head of the victim. Pain can be stabbing, throbbing, burning, squeezing, piercing, or drilling. It can move away from its starting location (usually behind the eye or the temple) and spread to the teeth, back of the head, and nose. A very evocative description of the utter devastation experienced during a cluster attack was provided by one patient: "Imagine waking up in the middle of the night and feeling a drill in your eye and feeling like somebody has pierced a hot metal rod through your neck and rammed it up into your brain. This is not a metaphor. This is what a cluster headache feels like."

Patients who also experienced an amputation, childbirth, breakthrough cancer pain, or severe burning describe the intensity of the pain of a cluster attack as at least comparable if not even worse. It's like the feeling of death, only you don't die, and the pain will start over again after a few hours. It's hard to imagine what it could mean to endure the pain of childbirth several times a day, every day for weeks or months—especially when no one can help you. Not even morphine can bring relief, and clusterheads know that ending up in an emergency room while you're screaming and writhing in agony isn't any better than dealing with the pain at home. It comes as no surprise that patients may start thinking that death is the only way to escape this torture. Although the conditions aren't fatal by themselves, cluster headache and migraine account for up to 80% of suicides in primary headaches. That's why this disorder is also referred as the "suicide headache." The name comes from a long history of patients taking the ultimate step to stop the pain.

During an attack, patients get restless, and still today we don't know if they writhe, scream, and run back and forth to cope with the immense pain or because of a much deeper neural mechanism. Yet there's no escape from the pain—as soon as it starts, it will reach its peak within 5–10 minutes, but the more it goes on, the worse it will get. Attacks usually last 45–90 minutes, but there are rattling recounts of patients enduring it for as long as three hours. And the horror isn't over when the attack ends. During a bad cluster, a much milder, TTH-like background pain known as "shadow" may linger for many hours after an attack is gone. In other words, what normal people call a "bad headache," one that makes them run for the nearest analgesic, is for clusterheads nothing but the background pain that will accompany them all day long. Just like hemicrania continua, the shadow of a cluster headache may last for weeks, months, or even years. And while this shadow never goes away, it is still much a more welcome sensation than being woken up at 3:00 a.m. by a devastating cluster attack.

Labeling this condition as a simple "headache" doesn't bring justice to the level of pain, disability, and generalized suffering that clusterheads must endure. Although the physical consequences of enduring such pain are obvious, the psychological ones are way too often underestimated. The anxiety of knowing beforehand that the attack is going to come at a certain hour is nearly as distressing as the pain itself and is certainly part of the agony. The majority of patients affected by this condition cannot live a normal life. Fear, stress, and depression become ghosts that will haunt their lives as they wait for the next cycle to come. Even pursuing a career or building a normal functioning family may represent significant challenges for individuals who must deal with excruciating and unbearable pain for half of their waking hours.

PAROXYSMAL HEMICRANIA

In paroxysmal hemicrania, the pain is usually severe in intensity and is described by patients as throbbing, burning, sharp, and stabbing. It is usually short-lived, lasting only 2–30 minutes, and is centered around the eye, temple, and forehead. While usually unilateral, pain can switch sides between attacks and in some instances spread across a larger region of the head. Attacks have a rapid onset and end up abruptly. They are associated with a broad range of autonomic symptoms such as conjunctival injection, sweating, tearing, runny nose, and flushing of the face or forehead on the same side of the headache. Restlessness or agitation during an episode is also frequently reported.

Attacks hit the patient many times a day, from 5 times a day up to 40 times a day, with an average of 11 a day. Mild background pain can persist between attacks. They come in bouts that last from seven days to one year, separated by remission periods that can last more than three months in episodic patients or less than three months in chronic patients. Onset is in adulthood, and the disorder may last indefinitely or spontaneously go into remission. Circadian mechanisms are likely involved in paroxysmal hemicrania due to its highly cyclic nature. In what seems to be the first case of this disorder ever documented, Johann Oppermann in 1747 described a 35-year-old woman suffering from recurring episodes of hemicranial pain that regularly affected her for 15 minutes every hour. No particular circannual recurrence characterizes symptomatic periods, although some patients can experience a seasonal preponderance.

Paroxysmal hemicrania attacks are usually spontaneous, but certain mechanical triggers also exist. Attacks can be primed by bending or turning the head and neck in some specific ways. Other triggers are also present in some patients and include stress or relaxation after stress, external pressure to the neck, alcohol, exercise, and cold or warm environments.

HEMICRANIA CONTINUA

In hemicrania continua, basal pain is a dull aching pressure similar to that of TTHs that occurs nearly always on the same side of the head and face. Pain ranges from mild to severe and is characterized by fluctuations where it increases in intensity up to three to five times per 24-hour cycle. The range of duration of exacerbations has no boundaries and varies from a few seconds to up to two weeks. While attacks tend to be more frequent at night, no circadian periodicity such as in cluster headache can be observed.

The nature of pain changes during the exacerbation phase, becoming more piercing, throbbing, and intense, generally paired with other highly debilitating symptoms such as nausea, vomiting, dizziness, and sensitivity to light and sounds. At least one autonomic symptom among those that are common for other TACs, such as eye redness, tearing, nasal congestion, miosis, and ptosis, is also present and is used for differential diagnosis purposes. During these exacerbation phases, hemicrania continua may mimic other primary and secondary headache disorders, with up to 70% of patients fulfilling the diagnostic criteria for migraine. Physical exertion, changes in sleep patterns, stress, or alcohol consumption can make the headache pain more severe in some patients.

SUNCT AND SUNA

SUNCT and SUNA are characterized by brief, sudden attacks of 5–240 seconds on one side of the head, with pain distributed in the forehead and temple regions, behind, and inside the eye, nose, and ear. Episodes are extremely painful and able to disrupt daily activities since they strike multiple times during the day. Pain is described as excruciating and stabbing, pulsating, electric, or burning in nature. In attacks of longer duration, the pain changes, following a sawtooth pattern characterized by multiple stabs. The number of attacks per day ranges between 3 and 200, with an average of around 60 times per day. Only a negligible percentage of attacks (less than 2%) occur at night. SUNCT and SUNA episodes are accompanied by local autonomic symptoms that include conjunctival injection, lacrimation, nasal congestion, forehead and facial sweating or flushing, eyelid edema, and ptosis.

The main difference between SUNCT and SUNA is the clinical presentation of the secondary autonomic symptoms. In SUNCT, both conjunctival injection (red eyes) and lacrimation on the same side of the headache should be present. In SUNA, one or both of these two symptoms are absent, and other autonomic symptoms may be present instead. SUNA attacks may also sometimes be longer, up to 10 minutes in total. It has been suggested that SUNCT syndrome may be a subset of SUNA; however, due to the rarity of these conditions, the small number of properly diagnosed patients does not allow for establishing a clear definition. In any case, SUNCT patients constitute the vast majority (more than 80%) of all reported SUNCT/SUNA cases.

Attacks are, for the most part, spontaneous, although several triggers that include a wide range of daily stimuli have been reported. SUNCT and SUNA triggers include many nearly unavoidable, everyday actions such as touching the scalp or face, chewing, eating, talking, brushing teeth, washing, showering, shaving, coughing, and blowing the nose. Exposure to light, strong smells, warm environment, smoke, and alcohol can also trigger an attack in some patients. Unlike trigeminal neuralgia, a disorder that also shares many similarities with SUNCT and SUNA, attacks can be triggered with no refractory period between them. Stress, fatigue, weather changes, and travels can worsen the bout, with more intense and frequent attacks.

TRIGEMINAL NEURALGIA

Trigeminal neuralgia is characterized by sudden, one-sided, severe pain that lasts from a fraction of a second up to two minutes. The intensity of pain can be physically and mentally incapacitating and is electric shock like, shooting, stabbing, or sharp in quality, but it can also become a more constant, aching, burning sensation. Attacks are usually sporadic and extremely painful, and they occur in quick succession, each volley lasting no more than two hours. Unlike with cluster headache, these episodes rarely occur at night while the patient is asleep. Attacks can be triggered by simple stimuli such as contact with the cheek or small vibrations. Even apparently innocuous actions such as eating, brushing teeth, shaving, drinking, talking, smiling, or being exposed to cold air or wind may trigger a painful attack of trigeminal neuralgia. Because of this, the condition is highly debilitating, as individuals affected may end up avoiding daily activities or social contacts for fear of the pain.

These episodes stop for a period of time and then return, usually becoming progressively more frequent, intense, and debilitating. Pain-free periods become shorter and shorter, and the condition becomes less responsive to the medication used to control the pain. Trigeminal neuralgia may evolve into an "atypical" form that is characterized by association with continuous or near-continuous aching of somewhat lower intensity between attacks. The pain is commonly associated with uncontrollable facial twitching, which is the reason why trigeminal neuralgia is also called tic douloureux. Because of the distribution of the trigeminal nerve, pain is often experienced along the jaw in the early stages of the disorder. Many patients wrongly assume they have a dental abscess, and they have a root canal performed. When the procedure brings no relief for the pain, they realize the problem is not dental related and seek out a neurologist.

HEADACHES CAUSED BY ACUTE SUBSTANCE USE OR EXPOSURE

The symptoms and clinical manifestations of headache associated with the use or exposure of substances are variable and depend on the individual substance as well as the quantity of that substance to which the patient was exposed. One of the most known types of headaches of this subtype is that which follows the consumption of acetaldehyde or alcohol, including alcoholic beverages, beer, wine, and distilled spirits. Alcohol consumption may result in acetaldehyde-accumulation metabolic acidosis and other changes in homeostasis, leading to dehydration, vasodilation, and general intoxication. Typical symptoms associated with the headache include nausea, dry mouth, drowsiness, impaired cognitive function, light sensitivity, general malaise, gastrointestinal issues, and irritability.

In nearly all headaches caused by acute substance use or exposure, pain is frequently bilateral, of pulsating quality, and of mild to moderate intensity, and it's aggravated by physical activity. The headache usually ends after the exposure is over, requiring no treatment and resolving spontaneously within 1–72 hours. In particular, a hangover can last for up to 24 hours, although it generally disappears within a much shorter time. In the case of carbon monoxide (CO), the severity varies with the severity of CO intoxication. Headache attributed to monosodium glutamate may be associated with its dose-dependent neuronal toxicity. For other substances, such as cocaine and histamine, headache may appear either immediately after exposure or after several hours in predisposed individuals. Some substances including alcohol or other vasodilators may trigger migraine or cluster headache attacks that follow the usual pattern of symptoms and clinical features.

HEADACHES ATTRIBUTED TO SUBSTANCE WITHDRAWAL

During substance withdrawal, headache is usually just a symptom of a larger syndrome that varies in relation to the substance to which the subject was originally addicted. Although caffeine is often used to ease the pain in some primary headache disorders, frequent consumption and/or addiction causes chronic vasoconstriction of the blood vessels of the brain. Withdrawal triggers rebound vasodilation and an unexpected increase in the blood flow of those areas. This sudden change in blood flow can cause throbbing headaches that usually start behind the eyes and then move up to other areas of the head (usually the front and sides). Their length and severity vary as the brain adapts to the increase in blood. Other symptoms of caffeine withdrawal include sleepiness, drowsiness, impaired cognitive functions, irritability and/or depression, lethargy, and constipation.

Prolonged use of substances such as alcohol, opioids, and benzodiaze-pines causes changes of specific receptors of the brain, spinal cord, auto-nomic nervous system, genitourinary system, and gastrointestinal tract. The body will slowly grow "accustomed" (addicted) to the presence of these substances, becoming desensitized to their effects and causing the overex-pression of these receptors. When the use of these substances is suddenly interrupted, these receptors that are now dependent upon the drug to function will start to malfunction, causing a plethora of symptoms that affect many organs and systems.

After quitting alcohol, depending on the severity of the substance abuse, headache is usually the first symptom that shows rather quickly. Alcohol withdrawal syndrome is associated with a broad range of different symptoms, ranging from anxiety to cravings, shakiness, mild fever, nau-sea, and vomiting. Headaches may also be present as a characteristic fea-ture of the post-acute-withdrawal syndrome (PAWS), a less acute condition that may persist for several weeks or months (sometimes years). Headaches may also develop after the interruption of daily consumption of opiate drugs for more than three months. However, they're usually a minor fea-ture of a larger withdrawal syndrome. Headaches resolve spontaneously within seven days in the absence of further consumption.

HEADACHES ATTRIBUTED TO HEAD OR NECK INJURIES

The clinical features of postconcussion headache may vary from one individual to another. In most cases, the clinical presentation simply mim-ics TTH, with mild- to moderate-intensity, migraine-like episodes occur-ring occasionally. A constellation of other acute neurological symptoms known as post-concussive syndrome may accompany the pain, ranging from nausea and/or vomiting to visual disturbances, dizziness and/or ver-tigo, tinnitus, muscle weakness, and tingling and/or numbness radiating down the shoulder, arm, hand, and/or fingers. These symptoms may linger for a much longer time after the original injury has completely healed, indicating an underlying disturbance of neurophysiological mechanisms of unknown origin. It has been postulated that, in some instances, a post-traumatic headache may represent the accentuation of another subclinical, infrequent, or undiagnosed preexisting primary headache rather than a new-onset headache directly linked to the trauma.

Postconcussion syndrome may also lead to the development of long-term or chronic psychological symptoms of undetermined origin, such as sleep disturbances, depression, anxiety, mood disturbances, behavioral changes, impaired memory and/or transient memory loss, concentration difficulty, and impaired libido. At the same time, sleep disturbances, mood disturbances, and psychosocial issues either caused by the same headache or by other factors may contribute to worsening the clinical features of the post-traumatic syndrome as a vicious cycle ensues.

CONCLUSION

Differentiating between headaches is often challenging due to the highly diversified clinical presentation of each individual case. Regardless of the diagnosis, individual patients must deal with their own individual head-ache, each one with its symptoms and triggers. In this chapter we analyzed a broad range of signs and symptoms that usually characterize each head-ache disorder, with "usually" being the key word here. In the next chapter, we will look at the other aspects of these very diversified disorders, in par-ticular, how they are diagnosed and how they are treated or managed.

5

Diagnosis, Treatment, and Management

They seemed to be selfish, these headaches, and yet they were not. The pain was real. No one could simulate such agonizing pain. Mr. Pritchard dreaded them more than anything in the world. A good one could make the whole house vibrate with horror.

—John Steinbeck

The life of a patient affected by a headache disorder is not a normal one. The more aggressive forms of this disease can have a tremendously negative impact on affected individuals' entire existence, limiting their ability to find and maintain a job, enjoy fulfilling relationships, and much more. A quick and accurate diagnosis and a proper treatment course are critical to ensure that these people can return to a normality as soon as possible, especially if a major headache disorder starts wrecking their lives while they're still very young (such as during childhood or early adolescence).

In this chapter we will explore how headaches are diagnosed as well as the challenges in constructing a proper differential diagnosis since this condition may manifest in so many different forms. We will understand how to determine whether some other underlying condition requiring urgent treatment is causing the headache. A broad overview of the many treatment alternatives, including both pharmacological and nonpharmacological ones, will also be provided.

THE CHALLENGES OF DIAGNOSING A HEADACHE DISORDER

Headache is among the most frequent medical complaints and one of the most common symptoms that primary- and secondary-care doctors evaluate in everyday practice. The high prevalence of this symptom and the vast heterogeneity of the different headache types and etiologies make differential diagnosis of headache disorders quite challenging. A differential diagnosis is the differentiation between different headache disorders that share similar clinical features. It is used to rule out other conditions that may cause the same symptoms. But what makes things even more complicated is that many headache disorders cause similar symptoms.

Although less than 1% of all headaches are actually life threatening, many of them can have a tremendous impact on the quality of life of untreated or misdiagnosed patients. Therefore, constructing a differential diagnosis without excessive evaluation is of the utmost importance. The co-occurrence of multiple headache disorders (such as tension-type headache [TTH] and migraine) is also commonly reported by patients, making the boundaries between the presentation of each disorder even more blurred. However, different kinds occur for a different reason, have a different origin and prognosis, and require different treatments and therapeutic approaches. Hence robust knowledge of the headache classification system (such as the *ICHD*-3) is a key aspect of the diagnostic process of a condition whose evaluation is mainly clinical in nature.

A careful history of the patient and a thorough physical examination are the first steps to determine the potential causes of each headache. Warning signals that raise red flags and prompt further diagnostic testing must be recognized—such as in the case of a suspected vascular disorder or head trauma. If no worrisome features that require further tests (e.g., diagnostic imaging or neurological examination) are detected in the history or examination of the patient, the primary syndrome must be diagnosed by assessing the clinical features. Traditional diagnostic tests (blood panels, laboratory studies, pathology, radiology) can only verify a secondary headache and are insufficient in verifying the diagnosis of a primary headache more often than not. Doctors must identify the unique characteristics of the acute attacks as well as their pattern and associated symptoms to make an accurate diagnosis. The single most important step in diagnosing headaches to determine if a headache is primary or secondary is asking whether the headache is new or old. New-onset headaches are frequently secondary, unless the patient is really young, while chronic ones with a well-defined pattern are more likely primary ones. Response to some specific therapies may also help in obtaining an accurate diagnosis (such as the response to verapamil in cluster headaches and to indomethacin in paroxysmal hemicrania).

However, things are rarely so simple. Although the clinical features of most headache disorders are diversified enough to eventually establish an accurate diagnosis, headaches can be unpredictable, sometimes occurring with subtle or unusual symptoms. While the diagnosis of secondary headaches can usually be confirmed through appropriate tests that assess the presence of the primary causative agent, there's no specific test to diagnose most primary headaches, such as migraines. When atypical features are present or the patient fails to respond to conventional therapy, the diagnosis should be revisited. Needless to say, a proper diagnosis is often obtained through trial and error and can take some time to be constructed.

SIGNS AND SYMPTOMS TO IDENTIFY A POTENTIALLY DANGEROUS HEADACHE

When a headache is a sign of a more serious disease or condition and is hence a secondary disorder, it is critical to identify it to provide adequate treatment right away. Early detection of these symptoms can make the difference between life and death. To sum it up, a headache can be the signal of a potentially life threatening, underlying issue when it is caused by:

- arteriovenous malformations or other abnormal connections between blood vessels in the brain.
- problems with circulation that prevent normal blood flow in certain areas of the brain (stroke).
- weakening of blood vessels within the head that can rupture causing an aneurysm.
- bleeding or collection of blood inside the brain (intracerebral hemorrhage) or in the tissues surrounding it (subarachnoid hemorrhage or hematoma, epidural hematoma) caused by trauma, concussions, carotid or vertebral artery dissection, or other spontaneous causes, such as hypertension or vessel fragility.
- brain injuries caused by accidents, trauma, or concussions.
- increased pressure inside the brain caused by the interruption of cerebrospinal fluid flow (acute obstructive hydrocephalus).
- emergency hypertensive crisis (high blood pressure).
- high pressure in the brain that is not caused by a tumor, although it appears to be (pseudotumor cerebri or idiopathic intracranial hypertension).
- brain tumors or other malignancies of the central nervous system.
- excess accumulation of fluid in the intracellular or extracellular spaces of the brain (brain edema) caused by carbon monoxide poisoning, altitude sickness, hypoxia, and other toxic or metabolic factors.

- infections of the brain (encephalitis), the spinal cord, and other parts of the central nervous system, caused by bacteria, parasites, protozoa, viruses, or fungi, such as meningitis or sepsis. They may or may not be associated with empyemas and abscesses (localized pockets of pus and other exudates that develop inside the brain or in the space between the tissues that cover it).
- noninfectious encephalopathies caused by metabolic or autoimmune disorders such as autoimmune encephalitis, hepatic encephalopathy, and posterior reversible encephalopathy syndrome (PRES).
- inflammation of or damage to the arteries that supply blood to the head, neck, and brain (temporal arteritis, giant-cell arteritis, or other types of vasculitis).
- serious pregnancy disorders, such as preeclampsia.

Promptly identifying the red flags for recognizing that a headache is potentially dangerous for the patient's health is a pivotal step during the diagnosis process. The essential job of the emergency clinician is to identify these features to distinguish one of the above-mentioned potentially threatening causes from the benign intrinsic ones of a primary headache disorder.

A headache usually requires urgent additional testing when:

- it is a new-onset headache. The patient never experienced it before, and it is severe enough to interfere with daily activities.
- it is a sudden-onset headache. The pain is extremely severe, persistent, severe, and/or explosive, and it reaches maximal intensity within a very short time frame (seconds or minutes).
- the headache develops acutely in close association with physical exertion or other physical activities such as running, lifting a weight, exercising, having sexual intercourse, and so forth.
- the attack is described by the patient as "the worst ever," even if the patient has regularly gotten headaches throughout life.
- there is a strong correlation between the onset of headache and a head or neck injury, trauma, or concussion.
- it is associated with one or more neurological symptoms, such as movement disorders, loss of balance, visual disturbances, slurred speech, confusion, or memory loss.
- the patient is over 50 years old and has a clinical history of cancer or cardiovascular, metabolic, or autoimmune disease.
- it becomes worse over the course of 24 hours or lasts more than a few days.
- it is associated with altered mental status or seizure.

- it is associated with a concurrent infection or symptoms that may indicate the presence of an infection, such as fever or stiff neck.
- the patient is under immunosuppressive therapy, is undergoing chemotherapy treatment, or has a compromised immune system (e.g., one affected by HIV).
- a brain tumor must be excluded, because the headache is associated with projectile vomiting, vomiting without nausea, and/or weight loss or because it is worse in the morning.

PHARMACOLOGICAL TREATMENTS

In clinical practice, the treatment paradigm has gradually shifted from a mainly suppressive treatment involving abortive therapy, to staunch the pain as it comes, toward an approach emphasizing prophylaxis and prevention. Today, although more holistic approaches tend to favor prevention in a broader sense (e.g., lifestyle changes, sleep hygiene, and dietary changes), pharmacological therapy of headache still remains a staple of headache treatment, especially for primary headache disorders. For some types of headaches, the currently available drugs can be insufficient to completely keep the disease under control, and sometimes the side effects can be somewhat of a concern. However, medicinal treatment has improved, by a significant margin, the quality of life of patients, especially those treated for the more aggressive disorders such as the trigeminal autonomic cephalalgias (TACs) and migraine.

Tension Headache

Simple analgesics and NSAIDs such as ibuprofen (400 mg), paracetamol (1,000 mg), and aspirin (500–1,000 mg) are the mainstays of acute TTH therapy, as they act as effective abortive agents in 75% of cases. Patients can self-manage their condition with OTC medications, but the efficacy of these drugs tends to decrease with increasing frequency of headaches. However, the use of drugs should be limited to episodic TTHs with a low attack frequency. It is critical to avoid frequent and excessive use of simple analgesics (more than 14 days a month) to prevent the risk of developing medication overuse or rebound headaches. The efficacy of simple analgesics can be increased by combination with caffeine (64–200 mg), oxycodone, or codeine, although there are no comparative studies examining the efficacy of combination with the latter two. However, patients using combination analgesics are at a higher risk of developing medication-overuse headache; therefore, such treatment should be recommended only in more severe cases.

For patients with frequent headaches or who respond poorly to abortive medications, preventive treatment should be considered. For example, in patients with chronic TTH linked with psychological issues such as anxiety or depression, simple analgesics are frequently ineffective, and non-drug treatments and prophylactic pharmacotherapy should be prioritized. Daily doses of the tricyclic antidepressant amitriptyline are the preferred choice due to the ability of this preventive agent to reduce pain and decrease muscle tenderness at the same time. Doses are usually gradually increased from a minimum of 10–25 milligrams per day up to 75–150 milligrams per day. However, the efficacy is modest, and side effects such as dry mouth, drowsiness, dizziness, obstipation (severe constipation), and weight gain may hamper therapy and compliance. Other nonpharmacological treatments such as posture improvement, dietary changes, sleep hygiene interventions, regular physical exercise, and relaxation techniques have proved to be effective as part of a headache treatment program.

Other antidepressants such as clomipramine, maprotiline, and mianserin have been reported to be more effective than placebo and can be used as second-line treatments when amitriptyline is not well tolerated. Antidepressants with action on both serotonin and noradrenaline, such as mirtazapine and venlafaxine, have been found to be effective at the same dosage needed for the treatment of depression. They may be used in selected cases, such as when there's a strong association between TTH episodes and this psychiatric condition.

Migraine

Pain-relief medications, or NSAIDs, are very often ineffective in patients with a high baseline migraine frequency who require higher and higher doses to glean even the slightest relief. Usually, specific medications such as the triptans are required to prevent a migraine attack or stop one in its tracks. For patients who experience fewer than two migraines per month or who use medications less than two days per week, abortive therapy is usually sufficient, unless the patient has developed tolerance to the medication. Serotonin receptor agonists (triptans) such as sumatriptan, almotriptan, rizatriptan, and zolmitriptan are administered in various formulations (standard or dissolution tablets, intranasal or sublingual spray, etc.) as first-line treatment options since they're effective and well tolerated by most patients.

The vasoconstrictive properties of triptans represent the main contraindication to these drugs. Although the incidence of cardiac problems is reported to be low, the potential for ischemic complications is still present, making serotonin receptor agonists contraindicated in patients with coronary artery disease, cerebrovascular disease, uncontrolled hypertension, rhythm disturbances, peripheral vascular disease, ischemic bowel disorders, and hemiplegic or basilar migraine. Other agents, such as ergot derivatives, barbiturate analgesics, opiates, caffeine, antiemetics, or a combination of more than one of these agents may be used to relieve a migraine attack.

Patients experiencing migraine attacks that are either too frequent (two or more per week), too long (lasting more than 48 hours), or unresponsive to abortive therapy may be candidates for preventive (prophylactic) therapy. The agents most commonly used for this purpose are the beta blockers (propranolol, atenolol, metoprolol, etc.), the tricyclic antidepressants (amitriptyline, nortriptyline, doxepin, desipramine), and some anticonvulsants (valproic acid, topiramate). Beta blockers are effective in approximately 70% of patients, and their use was well established by the 1970s. They are considered a drug of choice for migraine prevention, but they're not devoid of absolute contraindications (asthma, heart block, severe peripheral vascular disease), drug-drug interactions, and side effects (drowsiness, fatigue, cold hands, and weight gain, just to name a few). Albeit effective, antidepressants and anticonvulsants also share a similar range of side effects that some patients find difficult to cope with. Needless to say, a patient affected by chronic or frequent migraine has no choice but to accept the lesser evil.

Because of the significant level of suffering associated with migraine, desperate patients lacking proper diagnosis (and proper treatment) often cling to even the smallest form of relief. Due to the really high number of undiagnosed or misdiagnosed migraine patients (more than half), a relatively high percentage of them eventually end up hooked to high doses of self-administered OTC pain relievers, analgesics, and NSAIDs. Those unfortunate souls often develop medication-overuse headache (MOH) on top of an already frequent migraine, making their lives even more miserable. Other than increasing the risk of making the migraine become chronic, MOH can reduce efficacy of acute abortive therapy.

Cluster Headache

Treatment for cluster headache aims to stop the unbearable pain as quickly as possible (abortive treatment) as well as prevent it (preventive treatment). Since common painkillers and opioids are either ineffective or too slow to provide relief once the pain has started, acute treatment requires the use of rapid-action forms of administration. Typical abortive treatments include oxygen inhaled via face mask at medium- to high-flow rates (5–15 L/min.) and subcutaneous 6 milligram sumatriptan injections. For patients who cannot afford the high price of subcutaneous sumatriptan or have difficulties with self-injection, 5 milligram intranasal zolmitriptan is a good alternative. However, it is slower in providing immediate pain relief, requiring up to 15 minutes to be effective.

Prophylaxis is usually the preferred treatment, as episodic clusters that are not properly managed tend to have a higher risk of evolving into chronic forms. Verapamil, a calcium channel blocker represents first-line preventive treatment of cluster headache, although it requires a few days or weeks (usually 10–14 days) of treatment before it becomes effective in preventing episodes, and it requires slow titration of dosage for tolerability reasons. To provide effective prophylaxis during the transition period (before verapamil becomes effective), oral corticosteroids can be administered as bridge therapy for a limited period (one to three weeks, depending on the medication chosen) in selected patients. Prednisone is given at a starting dose of 60–80 milligrams daily; then it is reduced by 5 milligrams every day. Corticosteroids are also used to break cycles, especially in chronic patients. Occipital nerve block with both local infiltration of steroids and anesthetics for transitional therapy has also been tested in some patients, with mixed results. The ideal injection regimen for this type of treatment (e.g., which corticosteroid preparation, what form of application, or which dosage is the most efficient) has not been established.

Response to verapamil (120–480 mg per day) is sometimes used to ease the differential diagnosis since no other TAC or migraine responds to this drug. However, it is not always effective, with some patients reportedly using up to 1,200 milligrams per day (a nearly toxic dosage) to attain relief. Long-term verapamil use is also not devoid of concerning consequences. Approximately 19% of patients develop electrocardiogram abnormalities consisting mostly of prolonged PR intervals or right bundle branch blocks, with 4% of them developing complete heart block with junctional rhythms.

Subjects who do not tolerate the higher verapamil dosages or can't cope with the cardiovascular side effects may respond to medications used for epilepsy, such as topiramate, valproic acid, gabapentin, or lithium salts. Lithium at a dosage between 600 milligrams and 1,500 milligrams per day is the only agent approved for the prophylactic treatment of episodic cluster headache despite its serious side effects and the need for regular laboratory and plasma concentration monitoring. While ergot derivatives such as methysergide and ergotamine represented the first-line treatment in past decades, they are now infrequently prescribed due to their significant side effects and their risk of actually exacerbating the condition in the long term.

Prophylaxis should be continued for at least a month after the patient becomes asymptomatic, although a longer administration of the most effective medication may be required. To some extent, the length of the patient's previous clusters may serve as a guide, as longer clusters can require continued prophylactic treatment for up to three months (or more). Patient education, lifestyle changes, and the use of certain supplemental therapies (such as melatonin) are effective in reducing the frequency and severity of cluster bouts.

Case reports and recent studies suggest that the ingestion of some psychedelic or hallucinogenic substances such as psilocybin or LSD can reduce the pain of cluster headache and number of attacks per cycle or may even interrupt cycles. However, due to the highly controversial nature of this topic, we will discuss the use of psilocybin, LSD, and other psychotropic substances for people with cluster headaches and/or migraine in chapter 9.

Paroxysmal Hemicrania

In paroxysmal hemicrania, response to treatment is often used as a diagnostic criterion to differentiate this primary headache disorder from cluster headache. Paroxysmal hemicrania does, in fact, respond completely to the NSAID indomethacin at a dose of 25–150 milligrams per day. If the so-called indotest is used to determine if the patient is affected by this condition and to construct a differential diagnosis, then 50–100 milligrams indomethacin are given intramuscularly as a diagnostic test. This medication has an absolute effect on the symptoms but must be administered in several doses per day (usually three or four) due to its short half-life of four hours.

Unlike cluster headache, treatment with indomethacin cannot be suspended, so the goal is to determine the lowest effective dose that should be administered to achieve symptom control. Usually, a slow taper is trialed after an initial therapy of three to six months. Over time, most of the patients may reduce the dose of indomethacin required to maintain a pain-free state, and some are even able to withdraw completely.

Appropriate precautions such as the administration of ranitidine or proton pump inhibitors must be taken to prevent serious gastrointestinal and renal complications secondary to long-term use of indomethacin. About 20% of patients show side effects (mostly gastrointestinal ones) that lead them to treatment discontinuation. In those patients, other NSAIDs or cyclooxygenase-2 inhibitors, such as naproxen, aspirin, and diclofenac; or calcium channel blockers, such as verapamil and flunarizine, have been reported to be beneficial, although not to the full extent of indomethacin.

SUNCT and SUNA

Adequate management of SUNCT and SUNA remains an unsolved problem even today. These two TACs are known for their relative resistance to drug therapy, and still today, no first-line treatment or permanent cure is available. Since the attacks last a very short time and are frequent, abortive treatment is not an option, and no drugs are available to stop individual attacks.

Anticonvulsant or antiepileptic medications, such as lamotrigine, carbamazepine, gabapentin, and topiramate, can improve symptoms and provide some relief. However, they're associated with many long-term side effects, and their effectiveness is spotty at best. SUNCT may also respond to steroids for short-term treatment and verapamil for long-term reduction of symptoms and frequency of the attacks. However, these drugs are not as effective as in cluster headache. In particular, the calcium channel blocker may even worsen the symptoms in some patients.

Lamotrigine is the preferred treatment for SUNCT at doses of up to 300 milligrams daily, with up to 68% of patients responding positively to this medication. It acts by blockade of voltage-dependent sodium channel conductance, although other antifolate, antiglutamate, and antiaspartate actions have been suggested. SUNA may better respond to gabapentin, with a reported effectiveness of 60% in SUNA patients compared to only 45% in SUNCT patients. Topiramate, zonisamide, and carbamazepine represent a second-line therapy. If the patient is not responsive to pharmacological treatment, bilateral blockade of the greater occipital nerve, superior cervical ganglion opioid blockade, or botulinum toxin A infiltrated at four points around the orbit are all alternatives that can provide temporary or partial relief.

As for cluster headache, preventive treatments may require up to a few weeks before they are effective. To suppress attacks during this time frame, short-term transitional treatments that rapidly provide relief and decrease the flow of SUNCT/SUNA attacks are available. Intravenous lidocaine or subcutaneous infusion of lignocaine can be administered during the worst periods (the so-called SUNCT status) to achieve quick, although short-lasting, suppression of symptoms.

Hemicrania Continua

Patients with hemicrania continua may have suicidal thoughts or even attempt suicide because of the intolerable pain during severe exacerbations. The idea of unremitting torture that never ends, forcing the patient to endure it 24 hours a day for months is a nightmarish horror that some people can't stand for long. However, fortunately enough, hemicrania continua is characterized by complete response to therapeutic doses (25–300 mg) of indomethacin. The positive response to this drug is, in fact, a fundamental sine qua non criterion used in differential diagnosis. Unlike in paroxysmal hemicrania, in hemicrania continua the medication is gradually titrated from 25 milligrams three times per day up to 100 milligrams or until the patient gets complete relief. Response to the drug is complete in a few weeks, but the first effects become markedly noticeable immediately, with no delays such as in cluster headache or SUNCT/SUNA. Since long-standing painful conditions produce important morphological changes in the pain matrix, patients with a longer history of hemicrania continua may require more time before complete remission is achieved. Melatonin can, in any case, be administered, since it can either produce complete pain relief or at least allow up to 45% of patients taking indomethacin to reduce the dose.

Sadly, indomethacin must be taken daily and indefinitely to provide complete to near-complete relief of symptoms, since there's no cure. Another characteristic of hemicrania continua is the immediate reappearance of the symptoms if the drug is skipped and has a diagnostic value that is superior to even the indotest. More than 30% of patients cannot tolerate this treatment course in the long term due to the side effects of indomethacin: gastritis, gastric bleeding, allergy, high blood pressure, or exacerbation of asthma symptoms, among others. Since hemicrania continua is unexplainedly but exquisitely sensitive to indomethacin, these patients are forced to rely on less effective treatment. Gabapentin, topiramate, other NSAIDs such as COX-2 inhibitors (celecoxib and rofecoxib), and tricyclic antidepressants such as amitriptyline can all be used, but they do not offer a response of the same magnitude. Other drugs such as lamotrigine, lithium, naproxen, and paracetamol with caffeine have provided marked but partial effect on some patients. However, there's very little scientific literature available on the use of these alternative medications in hemicrania continua.

Trigeminal Neuralgia

Anticonvulsant drugs such as carbamazepine, oxcarbazepine, phenytoin, and gabapentin are the first line of treatment for trigeminal neuralgia. Carbamazepine is more effective than oxcarbazepine, but the latter has a better safety profile. The mechanism through which these drugs provide relief from pain is unknown and may be due to stabilization of hyperexcited neural membranes, inhibition of repetitive firing, or reduction of propagation of synaptic impulses. The dose is 300–800 milligrams per day, divided into two to three daily doses, and is usually lower than that required for the treatment of epilepsy. However, treatment becomes progressively less effective in providing relief over time due to the autoinduction of the drug itself, decreasing from approximately 80% to 50%.

Second-line treatment requires the administration of different drugs such as lamotrigine (400 mg/day), baclofen (40–80 mg/day), and pimozide (4–12 mg/day). These medications may be used either alone to switch therapy or as add-on therapy. Side effects include ataxia, dizziness, nausea, blurred vision, and skin rash. The rash can be severe and associated with fever or lymphadenopathy suggestive of Stevens–Johnson syndrome, which would require prompt discontinuation. Although a very slow titration of the dose will reduce the risk for these side effects to occur, many patients cannot tolerate an overly cautious and long titration phase. This is an inherent clinical dilemma that all health-care providers must face when treating trigeminal neuralgia. No bridge therapy is available such as in the case of cluster headache or SUNCT/SUNA, and the intense pain endured by the patient frequently compels a rapid medical response. However, a rapid dose escalation is not just risky but could also cause unpleasant dose-dependent side effects that may discourage the patient from trying that drug again.

Topiramate, valproate, clonazepam, and clonazepam can be used for patients who cannot tolerate first or second-line treatments, but literature on their effectiveness is somewhat limited. When medications become ineffective in treating the disorder, surgery may help control the pain. Surgical procedures such as microvascular decompression or percutaneous stereotactic rhizotomy are used to relieve nerve pain by either reducing the compression on the nerve or destroying the part of the nerve that is causing pain.

Medication-Overuse Headache

There is no universal consensus on how to treat MOH due to the broad variety of different clinical presentations available for this headache disorder. Patients with MOH are heterogenous, ranging from subjects affected by TTH, who overuse a single, highly accessible analgesic, to migraineurs suffering from several comorbid headaches with behavioral dependence and overuse of multiple medications. In most cases, it is also really hard to determine whether overuse of drugs is a cause or a consequence of the condition.

The preferred treatment for MOH is simply reduction of the dose and eventually discontinuation of overused medication, which is usually, but not invariably, sufficient to stop the pain. Simple advice to discontinue the overused medication can be sufficient in up to 70% of uncomplicated patients. Gradual tapering down of medication or bridge therapies may be necessary in case of physical dependence (benzodiazepines, opioids, and barbiturates) and in psychologically vulnerable patients. No withdrawal regime seems to be superior, but abrupt withdrawal is generally recommended in all cases where a tapered regime is not necessary, such as for patients overusing triptans or analgesics (even in combination with codeine). Other medications, such as antiemetics and neuroleptics, can be used to ease the withdrawal process by ameliorating abstinence-like symptoms. For the most severe types of headache disorder, or when the pain is too intense, another type of abortive medication—analgesics or intravenous administration of ergotamines—could be used in substitution (rescue medication).

The withdrawal process can initially lead to the worsening of headache and the appearance of drug withdrawal symptoms, including restlessness, agitation, difficulty sleeping, nausea, and gastrointestinal problems. These symptoms are transient (lasting up to a few weeks), but depending on the drug that was overused, they may be serious enough to require hospitalization for detoxification under medical supervision. Between 50% and 70% of patients who manage to discontinue the overused medication will revert to an episodic headache pattern that is usually associated with the preexisting headache.

Headaches Attributed to Head or Neck Injuries

The treatment of post-traumatic headache is symptomatic, as the disorder usually tapers off gradually within three to six months after the injury. Only 12% of patients with initial symptoms report having them after this time.

Each symptom is treated individually, with a preference for tricyclic antidepressants such as amitriptyline for their action on both the pain and the psychological symptoms. Treatment of post-traumatic headache is generally individualized in compliance with the standard therapeutic options of the headache disorders it mimics. For example, in the case of migraine-like episodes, the worst attacks can be treated with typical migraine medications such as the triptans.

HERBAL MEDICINE AND OTHER NATURAL REMEDIES

Many of the herbal remedies used to treat headaches have been described by a broad range of historical physicians such as Hippocrates, Pliny the Elder, Dioscorides, Galen, and Serenus Sammonicus. Nearly half of those we use even today were already included in the pharmacopoeia between the fifth century BCE and the second century CE, while others have been continuously used for over 2,000 years. According to a comparative study on plants used in Italian folk medicine, 78.4% of plant-based remedies contain active molecules or secondary metabolites that show anti-inflammatory, antinociceptive, and analgesic activities. Flavonoids, terpenoids, and phenylpropanoids may act as NSAIDs or possess inhibitory activities in the potential pathophysiological pathways triggering different types of headaches. Herbal remedies such as extracts of willow (*Salix spp.*) bark, ginger (*Zingiber officinale*), and honeysuckle (*Lonicera japonica*) may have found use in headache treatment due to their natural anti-inflammatory properties.

Others, such as *Hypericum perforatum* (St. John's wort), exhibited instead a more specific mechanism that inhibits several steps of the cascade of events associated with migraine's symptoms at the molecular level. According to a small study published in 2014, the benefits of ginger powder benefits could even be comparable to sumatriptan's in treating acute migraine, suggesting that the biological activity of this remedy can go well beyond a mere anti-inflammatory effect.

However, phytotherapic approaches in the treatment of headache is largely based on either traditional medicine or anecdotal knowledge. Only a minority of herbal drugs have had their safety and efficacy been studied adequately with well-controlled double-blind clinical trials. Namely, most studies focused only on a limited number of herbal remedies, including extract of St. John's wort, butterbur (*Petasites hybridus*), feverfew (*Tanacetun parthenium*), and a few others. However, despite their widespread use across history, very few plants found their effectiveness proved by clinical trials. For example, a Cochrane review of five large clinical trials on feverfew, one of the most known traditional remedies for migraine, showed little to no benefit for the majority of people who tried it.

There are many speculative reasons that may explain this difference between traditional use and clinical practice. For the most part, it's very hard to obtain consistent results due to the many variants involved in studying plants in clinical practice. Many phytochemical constituents found in medicinal herbs are present at very low concentrations that cannot be isolated and analyzed. Since plants are living organisms, characterizing all of the many metabolites present in the plant extract is often impossible. Apart from this, the commercially available products are often cultivated and may lack the properties that are found only in wild herbs. Plant constituents vary considerably in relation to environmental factors such as temperature, air humidity, availability of water and nutrients, sun exposure, and period of collection, as well as other factors involved in the manufacturing of the finished product (period, time, and method of collection; age of the plant; drying, storage; transportation, etc.). Some plant constituents may get destroyed during these processes or only be produced by the plant under specific circumstances (e.g., stress, droughts and specific amount of water and/or nutrients). Thus proper standardization of active principles, whose existence we may not even be aware of in the first place, may account for the wide variability of the therapeutic activity reported for many herbs.

Although some herbal remedies are associated with fewer side effects than pharmaceutical drugs are, the above-mentioned reasons represent a barrier that sometimes make phytotherapic approaches somewhat dangerous. For example, butterbur has been found so effective in the prophylaxis of adult migraines that both the American Headache Society and the Canadian Headache Society gave it a strong recommendation for its use in the prevention of migraine headaches. However, some preparations contain pyrrolizidine alkaloids, which display dangerous liver toxicity in humans. Therefore, not every butterbur product is safe for human consumption, and countries such as the United Kingdom and Germany have banned butterbur due to safety concerns.

NONPHARMACOLOGICAL MANAGEMENT OF HEADACHE

Nonpharmacological management of many types of headaches is widely used and is often considered for patients, either for prophylactic purposes (especially for TTH and migraine) or just to alleviate the symptoms and reduce the severity and frequency of the attacks (for some TACs and the most severe headache disorders). The efficacy of nondrug therapies including, among the most used, psychological treatments, EMG biofeedback (BF), acupuncture, relaxation training (RT), and physical therapy, is sparse, as is the scientific evidence surrounding them. Despite this, most of these approaches are highly valued for their relative simplicity, low cost, and absence of side effects normally associated with pharmacological therapies.

Many psychological treatments have proved to be effective in treating some types of headaches, especially TTH and migraine. The three main psychological approaches used for headache treatment are RT, BF, and cognitive behavioral therapy (CBT). RT helps reduce muscular tension that naturally arises over the course of a working day. The patient learns how to recognize and control this tension, thus relaxing those muscles that could trigger or at least worsen headache attacks. BF shares a very similar goal with RT but achieves it in a slightly different way. During a session of BF, one is provided with continuous feedback on the status and activity of one's muscles to recognize and control those that are in tension. In migraine, it also helps the patient understand and monitor other physiological processes associated with the experience of pain, such as changes in heart rate and blood pressure.

CBT helps the patient identify thought and mental patterns that could generate stress and aggravate attacks. Subjects learn to challenge these thoughts through coping techniques that help them adapt their behaviors. The exact degree of effect of psychological treatments cannot be precisely determined since it's hard to make a reliable comparison with placebo procedures. The headache index is reduced by nearly one-third for all three strategies, but the absence of documented guidelines to standardize them means that individual differences can be significant (e.g., how much that patient is affected by psychological problems or affective distress).

The most used nonpharmacological treatment of headache is physical therapy, whose aim is still to reduce muscle contractions. However, this time the patient should achieve this goal through self-improvement of posture, massages to relax muscles, exercise programs, electrical or ultrasound stimulation, and hot/cold packs. The effectiveness of these treatment strategies has never been properly evaluated by reproducible clinical trials, but given their relative simplicity and high tolerability, they can be recommended to allow a certain degree of self-management.

The use of acupuncture in TTH and migraine has yielded conflicting results, especially since very few randomized clinical trials have compared the effectiveness of standard-of-care acupuncture to sham therapies. In general, there's some evidence that minimal acupuncture is better than no treatment and that laser acupuncture is a reliable alternative while acupuncture-like electrical stimulation is not. Studies that compared the effect of verum acupuncture to sham acupuncture and standard therapy showed a reduction in number of migraine days with reference to baseline, with no difference between the three alternatives. This suggests that the biological effect of this therapeutic strategy may not depend on the positioning of the needles themselves.

Surgical Therapies

In recent years, surgery has emerged as an effective alternative treatment for chronic patients with restricted medical options (such as people who cannot tolerate standard treatment or for whom it is contraindicated) or intractable primary headaches. Chronic temporal headaches, such as TTH and migraine, as well as more severe primary headaches, such as cluster headache and SUNCT/SUNA, can be treated with invasive surgical procedures in medication-refractory cases. Although surgery usually provides immediate relief, there are chances of recurrence, which suggests deeper pathophysiological mechanisms that go beyond mere nerve inflammation.

Plastic surgeons noticed that some chronic migraineurs found partial relief from their headaches after some cosmetic procedures, such as forehead lift. Severe headaches are worsened or sometimes caused by muscle spasms or dilated blood vessels exerting pressure on the branches of the trigeminal nerve located on the side of the head. This compression ultimately leads to inflammation of the nerves and membranes surrounding the brain, causing many of the symptoms associated with primary headaches. Surgery seeks to relieve pressure on these "trigger sites" by either releasing muscle fibers or desensitizing nerves by disconnecting them in order to reduce headache pain. To date, five main areas have been identified as trigger sites—namely, frontal, anterior temporal, posterior temporal, occipital, and rhinogenic (when headaches are caused by hypertrophied turbinates or deviated nasal septum).

To ascertain whether a patient is a good candidate for peripheral neurolysis, surgical decompression, or ablative procedures, botulinum toxin has to be injected into trigger sites to temporarily block muscle activity, or local anesthetics are instilled to temporarily block the involved nerve. Continuous pain relief for 6–12 weeks indicates an appropriate candidate for the surgery. Neurolysis is obtained by applying a physical or chemical destructive agent to a nerve in order to interrupt neural transmission permanently. The exact type of surgical procedure required depends on the trigger site. For example, for cluster headache, radiofrequency thermocoagulation (RTFA) of the sphenopalatine ganglion is the most commonly used surgical neurotomy technique to destroy painful nerves with heat. Adverse events with radiofrequency procedures include facial dysesthesias, corneal sensory loss, motor weakness, keratitis, and anesthesia dolorosa.

Gamma knife radiosurgery is a less invasive technique where the trigeminal nerve is injured with a beam of radiation. The procedure is done on an outpatient basis and has shown promising results in treatment of refractory cluster headaches with low complication rates. However, very few medical institutions have gamma knife capabilities, and more studies are necessary to investigate the relapse rates (which seem to be high), long-term effects, and complications of this procedure. Microvascular decompression is another, more invasive surgical procedure used in cluster headache and trigeminal neuralgia that involves craniectomy. During the procedure, a vascular loop compressing a nerve is removed to restore normal anatomy. However, the success rate is lower than 50% in long-term follow-up studies.

CONCLUSION

This chapter explained the complexities of properly assessing the exact type of headache that is affecting the patient. We also identified the signs that suggest the headache can be an underlying symptom of a potentially life-threatening condition or disorder. Lastly, we explored all the currently available standards of treatment—both pharmacological and nonpharmacological—for headaches. In the next chapter, we will address the most common comorbidities associated with headache disorders, the psychosocial and economic impact of headache in patients' lives, their chances of recovery, and long-term health outcomes and prognosis.

6

Long-Term Prognosis and Potential Complications

That no one dies of migraine seems, to someone deep into an attack, an ambiguous blessing.

—Joan Didion

Primary headaches are generally described as relatively benign conditions and are often underestimated by the general public, mostly because they are episodic, do not cause death, and are not contagious. However, living with a severe headache means having to endure many challenges, as these conditions come with a substantial personal burden in terms of pain, disability, and reduced quality of life. Primary headaches also have significant societal costs that translate to countless working days lost across the world. Recall that primary headaches are frequently accompanied by many comorbidities and can have serious psychological consequences. In this chapter, we will look at all these less objective but no less important aspects of how severe headaches affect the psychological, social, and economic aspects of patients' lives, as well as the extended outlook for them in both the short and long term.

COMORBIDITY

In patients affected by a headache disorder, comorbidities are defined as co-occurring conditions that are present as separate illnesses at a frequency greater than would be expected by chance. There are many reasons why understanding comorbidities is vital to improve the understanding of a disease and its management. Since they are interrelated with the primary disorder, they help shed a light on the possible pathophysiology of the headache disorder, which is particularly important for most primary headaches, such as migraine and cluster headache, whose intrinsic mechanisms are still unclear. The identification of comorbidities could be instrumental in recognizing common underlying genetic mechanisms of diseases to develop new, targeted molecules for treatment or to inform a more efficient treatment. For example, if a patient has both migraine and depression, an antidepressant can be favored as preventive medication to address both conditions with a single drug. Comorbidities also substantially contribute in diminishing the quality of life in patients who are already struggling with a major headache. First, they often complicate diagnosis, lead to underdiagnosis, and can limit treatment options. For example, a cardiovascular comorbidity may limit the ability to use triptans.

However, at the same time, it is important to remember that the high rate of misdiagnosis associated mostly with migraine and trigeminal autonomic cephalalgias (TACs) could be the reason for many additional conditions wrongly perceived as comorbidities. For example, in patients later diagnosed with cluster headache, the numerous previous diagnoses of depression, deviated septum, or dental/temporomandibular joint problems may not be true comorbidities but perhaps reflect just inaccurate diagnoses of the cause of their unilateral head pain.

Probably the most common comorbidities with primary headache disorders are psychiatric disorders, likely due to the significant burden exerted by these conditions on the psychological well-being of patients affected. Roughly 37% of chronic migraine patients suffer from a mental disorder, with the most common ones being depression, bipolar disorder, and anxiety. It should be noted that the risk of anxiety and depression has not been fully investigated during the different phases of cluster headache (active bout vs. remission). Some studies, in fact, pointed out how the cyclical nature of cluster headache might apply to the psychiatric comorbidities experienced by this group of patients. In any case, stress and psychiatric comorbidities can influence the disease burden well beyond the obvious negative effect on the quality of life they have on patients with a headache disorder. Anxiety and depression tend to complicate the management of the condition, increase the direct and indirect costs of migraine, and increase the risk of evolving it into a chronic form.

Therefore, optimal management of psychiatric comorbidities is critical to improve adherence to and effectiveness of headache therapy, ultimately improving quality of life.

Among the anxiety disorders, the ones most commonly associated with migraine and cluster headache are generalized anxiety disorder, obsessive-compulsive disorder, and panic disorder. The risk of suffering from bipolar disorder is about two times higher in migraine patients, and post-traumatic stress disorder (PTSD) also appears to be particularly frequent. Lifetime prevalence and onset of panic disorder are higher in subjects with migraine and other severe headaches as well.

The risk of depression in migraineurs is two to four times greater than in nonmigraineurs, and the association appears to be even stronger in patients with the aura subtype, patients affected by chronic forms, and patients with marked allodynia. Depressed migraine patients also seem to be more likely to not respond to treatment and to have a higher chance of suffering from abuse of symptomatic drugs and medication-overuse headache (MOH). More generally, patients with chronic daily headaches have statistically significant higher levels of alcohol consumption, and their physical pain is reflected in their psychological state. They frequently present with a sense of emptiness, sadness, and pain that may be visible even in their facial expressions.

Although scientific evidence available so far is insufficient to show a clear causal relationship between psychiatric disorders and primary headaches, neuroimaging studies show alterations in the brain areas involved in the emotional response to pain. Migraineurs' emotional reactions to pain, light, noise, and odors may be abnormally stronger than those of people not affected by this condition. In patients affected by depression and other psychiatric disorders, the connectivity between affective-motivational areas and the areas responsible for discriminating sensory stimuli is also increased, suggesting a possible common pathogenetic link.

Many studies found an association between migraine and cardiovascular problems. More specifically, severe headache pain is associated with increased risk of peripheral artery disease, hypertension, and high cholesterol, while migraine with aura is associated with ischemic stroke. On top of that, approximately one-third of chronic migraine patients suffer from hypertension and hyperlipidemia, and 9.6% of them are diagnosed with coronary heart disease. Interestingly enough, the risk of cardiovascular diseases is doubled in migraine with aura patients only if they carry a certain DD/DI genotype, although more studies are needed to confirm and investigate this association. In contrast, no association was found for angina and myocardial infarction. The frequency and severity of chronic headaches and migraine attacks are increased up to fivefold in obese patients. In particular, the severity and frequency of headache attacks progressively increase with increments in body weight categories, from normal weight, to overweight, obese, and morbidly obese.

Migraine and other severe headache disorders are associated with sleep disorders, including insomnia, restless leg syndrome, parasomnias, and sleep apnea. Other than worsening other underlying comorbidities such as cardiovascular diseases and psychiatric disorders, poor sleep quality seemingly affects the frequency and severity of headache attacks. The bidirectional relationship between migraine, cluster headache, and sleep problems seemingly suggests the existence of a common underlying pathophysiology and shared anatomical structures within the brain.

Migraine is linked with epilepsy as much as epilepsy is linked to migraine. The presence of one of these disorders increases the likelihood of the other, possibly because the state of neuronal hyperexcitability that characterizes both conditions can be due to a common pathogenetic mechanism. When a subject is affected by epilepsy and a primary headache disorder, therapy with medications effective for both conditions represents the optimal therapeutic choice. Several chronic pain disorders, such as fibromyalgia, arthritis, neuropathic pain, and noncephalic pain, were reported to be associated with migraine, trigeminal neuralgia, and other forms of severe headache pain. The intensity of severe headache can be associated with an increased risk of allergy and psoriasis, and many primary headache disorders are 1.5 times more likely among those with asthma, hay fever, and chronic bronchitis than those without.

For cluster headache, a statistically significant association between the disorder and sinus or dental problems has been found, as well as a significant increase in smoking habits. Interestingly enough, cluster headache patients do not show an increased risk of alcohol consumption as migraineurs, probably due to the negative effect of this substance on the severity and frequency of cluster attacks. However, as we already pointed out, deviated septum and dental or temporomandibular problems can just represent previous tentative diagnoses of their unexplained unilateral head pain. Patients with cluster headache are also at increased risk for depression, anxiety, and self-injury or suicide attempts during attacks. However, this risk is higher in chronic or undiagnosed/misdiagnosed forms as well as those forms that are unresponsive to treatment. On the other hand, the prevalence of diabetes is significantly lower in patients with cluster headache, so much that some authors suggested a potentially protective action of this endocrine disorder against the expression or development of cluster headache. Notably, a certain overlap between cluster headache and migraine has been reported, with the latter being present as a comorbidity in 10%–16.7% of patients. Up to half of patients with cluster headache experience symptoms that are shared by migraine, such as nausea, vomiting, phonophobia, and photophobia. Because the two conditions also share common triggers, a possible genetic link, and a good therapeutic response to the same class of drugs (triptans), an underlying common mechanism can be hypothesized. Coexisting migraine may also independently influence the risk for psychiatric comorbidities in cluster headache patients, further increasing the disease burden.

Vitamin D deficiency is also very common in patients with cluster headache, and a possible link with serum vitamin D–level seasonal variations is suggested by the increase in frequency of headache attacks during the autumn and winter, as experienced by many subjects. Although the exact relationship between vitamin D deficiency and headache still remains quite enigmatic, supplementation of vitamin D has been reported to be beneficial to certain patients.

The vast majority of contemporary literature on headache disorders focuses on migraine and cluster headaches, with only a few studies examining the comorbidities of other primary headaches, such as tension-type headaches (TTH). A high prevalence of psychiatric and psychologic disorders has been found in patients with TTH, especially in those suffering from the chronic forms. The frequency and severity of attacks seem to be associated with increased affective distress and maladaptive coping.

SOCIOECONOMIC IMPACT AND DISABILITY

Headache disorders are among the most common disorders of the nervous system and are associated with a significant personal and societal burden in terms of pain, disability, reduced quality of life, and financial costs. With nearly half of the adult population suffering from a headache episode at least once within one year, headache disorders are among the most prevalent disorders worldwide. This estimate is probably nowhere near to representing the real size of the headache burden, since it is known that only a minority of patients worldwide receive an appropriate diagnosis by a health-care provider. Nevertheless, headache burden is globally underrecognized and underestimated in scope and scale, possibly because of the nonfatal nature of headaches and the fact that they seldom result in permanent or objective disability.

Collectively, all headache disorders represented the third cause of disability in people under 50 years of age in the Global Burden of Diseases, Injuries, and Risk Factors (GBD) 2015 report. In 2016 alone, nearly three billion people had a migraine or TTH. Migraine and TTH caused a total of 52.3 million years of life lived with disability (YLDs), with migraine contributing much more significantly to this number, with 45.1 million YLDs. Together, TTH and migraine accounted for 6.5% of all YLDs, reaching a maximum of 11.2% of YLDs among women ages 15–49 years. This means that the social impact, in terms of reduced productivity, of these disorders is huge, since they are especially troublesome in the productive years.

TTHs are the third most prevalent disorder worldwide after dental caries and latent tuberculosis infection. Headache disorders not only cause suffering for the individuals affected but they also have a substantial social and economic impact in modern society. This burden includes both direct costs associated with the use of health-care resources (drugs, emergency room visits, diagnostic procedures, physician visits, etc.) and indirect societal costs associated with reduced efficiency. The cost of migraine and its treatment is estimated between $13 to $17 billion in the United States, roughly one-tenth of which ($1.5 billion) is for medication. Indirect costs (work loss and reduced productivity) account for the vast majority of the annual per-person cost of migraine. Both diagnosed and undiagnosed migraine has a negative impact on worker productivity. Every working day, more than 100,000 people are absent from work or school because of migraine alone. Migraine and chronic headache have been found to be the second most frequently identified cause of short-term absence (47%) for nonmanual employees. In the United Kingdom, migraine causes 25 million working or schooldays to be lost, and roughly the same number are lost due to TTH and MOH combined. On average, a male patient with migraine loses 1 workday, 1 housework day, and 1 day of social time per month, while female patients lose 1 workday, 2 housework days, and 1.5 days of social time per month. In most cases, migraines can lead to a reduction in work or school productivity greater than 50%. In stressful work environments, the impact of migraine is even more evident and, for obvious reasons, costs are higher for chronic headaches than for episodic ones. Lost productivity includes both absenteeism, disability, and presenteeism (attending work while ill). In particular, migraine-related presenteeism costs represent nearly 90% of the total costs associated with the condition. Interestingly enough, most studies found that workplace migraine-intervention programs focused on prevention and symptomatic treatment could significantly reduce the loss in worker productivity. Appropriate therapeutic strategies and the help of health-care professionals and occupational health clinics have a profound impact in reducing the burden of migraine for employees and employers alike. The individual cost for migraine ranges from $2,649 per year to $8,243 per year for the chronic form in the United States. In Europe, due to the partly public nature of the various national health-care systems, the cost is lower yet still significant, ranging from €746 per year to €2,427 per year for the chronic form.

An aspect that is often neglected is that severe or recurrent headache attacks do not just affect productivity but also have a profound impact on an individual's life as a whole. To put things in perspective, on average, patients with migraine spend 5.3% of their lives experiencing attacks.

Many limitations forced upon the lives of patients amount to days with reduced household and leisure activities, as well as limitations in terms of being able to care for and deal with their children, all of which contribute to making their lives even more miserable. There are also many other "intangible" aspects that have never been properly accounted for by most studies, such as time spent searching for proper care or the activities missed or plans canceled due to the fear of having an attack. Approximately half of patients with migraine state that the disorder had a negative impact on their social or family life. This can be summed up in terms of missing important events (birthdays, weddings, other social events), avoiding making commitments, not participating in all activities/hobbies they used to, having negative effects on sex life, being stopped from engaging in sports activities or exercise, and experiencing negative feelings (frustration, hopelessness, guilt about the impact the disease has on their family).

PSYCHOLOGICAL CONSEQUENCES OF HEADACHE

Pain, autonomic signs, and all the other physical symptoms alone are insufficient to account for the full extent of disability and psychological discomfort experienced by a patient with a severe headache disorder. In this chapter, we outlined the broad range of negative feelings that are often associated with living with a headache. Although psychiatric disorders such as anxiety, depression, or suicidal thoughts are described as known comorbidities of headache disorders, it is clear that the number of patients who receive such a diagnosis only represent the most extreme cases. Yet they are only the tip of the iceberg among a much more significant number of patients who must endure a broad range of negative feelings that have a tremendous impact on their lives and that certainly contribute to the overall burden of the disease. After all, chronic headaches can have a devastating and disruptive effect on normal living. Other than the pain itself, sufferers may have to face prejudices in the workplace, job loss, social ostracism, and disruption to personal relationships.

The link between severe headache disorders and depression can lead to many other symptoms such as reduced self-confidence, low self-esteem, and weight gain. Patients affected by nontrivial headaches frequently feel like they are always lacking the energy to complete the tasks of daily living, have difficulty concentrating on tasks, have to cancel plans, and cannot participate in family activities. Such constant interference can ultimately make them feel hopeless, helpless, frustrated, angry, or even scared. In a never-ending loop of negativity, the frequency, duration, and intensity of headache attacks can increase due to their poor sleep, depressed mood, pain catastrophizing, and perceived loss of control over the disease, which can precipitate migraine. And the more severe the impairments in functioning and quality of life, the worse the overall mood and psychological well-being of the subject will be, establishing a vicious cycle that is hardly accounted for during treatment.

Most of the actual scientific discussion on headache focuses more on the neurophysiological and neuroanatomical aspects of the disease than on the effects on patients. However, headache is characterized by pain, which, although subjective, is unquestionably unpleasant and therefore a negative emotional experience. It is central to remember that, besides treating the disease as detached entity, headache patients are human beings, and they are living with the disease that needs treatment. Surveys report that many patients feel that physicians fail to understand how their condition interferes with their life, showing how communication about severe headaches is frequently incomplete. Psychological interventions such as biofeedback and psychotherapy can be useful adjuncts to pharmacological therapy, but they're also important in helping patients manage their lifestyles, reduce their stress, and ultimately improve the quality of their lives.

THE DIFFERENCES BETWEEN MEN AND WOMEN

A significant gender disparity exists in migraine and other headache disorders, with men being affected differently than women at the biological, physical, social, and psychological levels. Migraine, for example, affects approximately three times as many women as men—18% of women and 6% of men—in the United States. The difference between men and women in migraine prevalence is so pronounced that the disease has become feminized, and male subjects with migraine are now at risk for being underdiagnosed and undertreated. This preponderance emerges at puberty, with females having a 1.5-fold greater risk of headaches and a 1.7-fold greater risk of migraine than male children and adolescents have. As a result, women account for about 80% of the $78 billion in migraine-associated economic costs in the United States. However, for some primary headache disorders, this prevalence may be different. For example, for TTHs, there's no difference in prevalence between men and women, while cluster headache affects men more than women by a factor of roughly three to one.

The explanation for this disparity is still undetermined, although many hypotheses have been proposed, including genetic factors, fluctuations in sex hormones, and differences in response to stress and pain perception. For example, a correlation with female sex hormones has been identified since menstruation-related migraine affects 55% of women, and migraine's severity and frequency are reduced in most women during pregnancy and after menopause. Some studies also found that migraine attacks last longer, are more painful, and cause more severe disability in female subjects on average. Higher levels of estrogen have been proposed as a potential explanation for this difference, since it can elevate pain levels during the menstrual cycle, although the women's lower pain threshold as well as the male cultural attitude toward machismo and enduring pain may explain this difference. At the same time, men with migraine are more likely than their women counterparts to go into partial or total remission. Other psychological and sociocultural factors may play a role in the observed differences between males and females. For example, the risk factors for transition to chronic migraine include conditions that are more commonly reported in women than in men, such as depression, anxiety, and obesity. Also, traumatic childhood experiences and intimate partner violence can increase the risk for migraine, and rates of sexual violence, harassment, and assault are higher in women.

Even the triggers flaring up an attack seem to be different, with males often reporting physical exertion and alcohol as migraine triggers while women report weather changes and smells. Lastly, while women are more sensitive to perfumes and odors during an attack, men are more sensitive to light and are more likely to report photophobia as a symptom. Comorbid conditions also seem to be different between sexes, with women reporting 11 comorbidities versus 5 for men, on average. Comorbid conditions more frequently reported in women include anxiety, depression, fibromyalgia, endometriosis, and restless legs syndrome, whereas in men, reported comorbidities include obesity, coronary thrombosis, diabetes, epilepsy, and kidney stones. However, data are somewhat contradictory, and further studies are needed. Migraine in women can also represent a risk factor for preeclampsia, a vascular disorder of pregnancy characterized by high blood pressure, vasospasm, and organ damage. Preeclampsia is the leading cause of death among pregnant women. An association between preeclampsia and migraine has been found, particularly in female patients whose migraine attacks were exacerbated during pregnancy, leading to adverse cardiovascular outcomes.

MIGRAINOUS INFARCTION AND OTHER MIGRAINE COMPLICATIONS

Despite being an otherwise benign condition, migraine, especially the variety with aura, is a well-known risk factor for cerebral infarction (stroke). Sometimes a migraine attack (predominantly with aura) can be associated with signs of a silent infarction. In particular, the term "migrainous infarction" (or "migrainous stroke") is used when an ischemic stroke occurs in correspondence with migraine aura symptoms that gradually worsen and cause serious neurological changes. More specifically, the *ICHD*-3 provides the definition of migrainous infarction as "one or more migraine aura symptoms associated with an ischemic brain lesion in the appropriate territory demonstrated by neuroimaging."

If the symptoms of a migraine aura last for more than 60 minutes, a migrainous infarction could be underway. The patient may also have experienced more severe aura symptoms in the month prior to the cerebral infarction. Migrainous infarction may also occur in patients who never experienced a migraine aura, although it's significantly less common, affecting only 20% of these patients.

Migraine itself represents an independent risk factor for cardiovascular diseases, increasing the risk for acute myocardial infarction, angina, and stroke by 1.5 times, and mortality by cardiovascular diseases by 1.37 times. Since this risk is mostly linked to cerebral ischemia, migrainous infarction is one of the most dangerous complications of migraine. Patients at a greater risk for developing migrainous infarction are women under the age of 45 who experience migraine with aura, especially if they use oral contraceptives and/or smoke tobacco. Migraine with aura presents a relative risk of 2.16 for cerebral ischemia, which can be higher in children and in patients with a higher frequency of migraine attacks. Migrainous stroke is a serious complication of migraine, accounting for 0.5–1.5% of all ischemic strokes and 10% of strokes in younger patients.

The pathogenesis of migrainous infarction is still unclear, although it is believed that the reduced blood flow and the biochemical and hemodynamic changes associated with cortical spreading depression (CSD) may play a central role. How migraine does increase the risk of cerebral ischemia is also debated, and various theories have been proposed:

1. Many of the drugs used to treat migraine such as triptans, dihydroergotamine, and ergot derivatives have vascular effects, which may ultimately increase the risk for cerebral ischemia.

2. Patients affected by migraine may have a genetic predisposition toward hyperactivity of vessels.

3. Migraine may increase the risk of atheromatous plaque formation by causing an endothelial dysfunction which leads to increased coagulation, tissue hyperproliferation, and subchronic inflammatory states.

4. Migraine aura could increase platelet activation even during headache-free periods, thus increasing the risk of developing thrombosis. Because of this, thrombolytic agents and anti-aggregation drugs such as aspirin are often administered as a treatment option for migrainous infarction.

When aura is prolonged for several hours or days, in the absence of radiographic evidence of cerebral infarction, a diagnosis of *migraine with persistent aura* (another rare complication) must be made. Symptoms of migraine with persistent aura are often bilateral and may last for months or years. If the attack itself, rather than just the aura symptoms, lasts for more than 72 hours, another highly debilitating complication known as *status migrainosus* may be occurring. Status migrainosus is often associated with medication overuse, highlighting the importance of adequate prophylaxis in migraine management. Poor acute treatment may, in fact, lead to chronic or complicated migraine quite frequently.

Another rare complication of migraine is *migraine aura-triggered seizure*, also widely known as *migralepsy*, a condition where a patient experiences a seizure within one hour of a typical migraine aura attack. Due to the high comorbidity of migraine and epilepsy and the similarity in symptoms and treatments of the two conditions, it has been postulated that the two may share the same pathophysiology. However, migralepsy is a rare phenomenon, and the true nature of the association between migraine and epilepsy is still largely unclear. It is quite possible that migralepsy can be simply a very severe case of migraine that precipitates into a seizure attack. In any case, since most antiepileptic agents are equally effective in controlling seizures and preventing migraine, these medications are often used as the drug of choice for the treatment of migralepsy.

LONG-TERM PROGNOSIS AND HEALTH OUTCOMES OF HEADACHE

Many different psychological, clinical, social, and demographic factors may affect prognosis and treatment outcome in patients with a primary headache disorder. Comorbidity with psychiatric disorders or other negative psychological or lifestyle factors such as high stress, smoking, alcohol consumption, low headache management self-efficacy, medication overuse, and poor sleep quality are generally associated with worse outcomes. Other factors, such as high frequency and severity of attacks, obesity, or presence of allodynia in migraine, are also predictive of worse health outcomes.

More in general, headaches are associated with a benign prognosis, since they usually go into complete or at least partial remission. In people ages 40 and above, the severity and frequency of migraine and cluster headache attacks generally tend to diminish as the patients grow older. Women may experience a partial or total remission during or after pregnancy and menopause, since hormonal levels can be a factor. More than one-third of patients go into complete remission after 15 years of suffering migraines. Although cluster headaches generally tend to be a lifelong condition, remission periods tend to get longer with age, and bouts are often less severe. For severe headache disorders, the benefit of remission goes beyond symptom reduction and may lead to reduced headache-related disability.

Sadly, although the clinical presentation of most headaches shows clear age-dependent changes, there is no systematic review of how the symptoms evolve during the life span. Migraine attacks tend to have a significantly shorter duration during childhood, with more prominent paroxysmal symptoms, such as vomiting, abdominal pain, or vertigo. In contrast, migraine attacks tend to be devoid of autonomic signs during old age, with pain occurring more often bilaterally or in the neck area. These variations may be due to age-related changes in the reactivity of the cerebral blood vessels that cause pain to distribute more globally across the head, together with a decline of the activity of the autonomic nervous system, which may account for the reduction of autonomic symptoms. In other headache disorders such as cluster headache and TTH, instead, the age-dependent differences tend to be less distinct. In female children with pediatric onset of cluster headache, the headache seems to have a more frequent chronic course, while in males, attacks have a higher frequency and longer duration. Eventually, cluster headache tends to fade off with time, with elderly patients generally reporting less frequent cluster bouts than adults do. However, the clinical presentation of attacks seems to remain the same, albeit with less severe symptoms and pain. This may be the consequence of changes in reactivity of the cerebral and extracerebral blood vessels to the hypothalamic stimuli associated with natural brain aging.

Age at onset of headache seems to be a relevant factor as well. Some short-term follow-up studies found that a significant number of patients who received a diagnosis of headache during childhood will improve or remit in 60%–80% of cases in the subsequent 10 years. Despite the apparently favorable outcome, however, childhood headaches represent the third most frequent cause of school absenteeism. On top of that, other studies that examined the persistence of headache into adulthood found that a much larger number of patients who received a diagnosis of pediatric headaches continue to have headaches in the ensuing 20 years. This is particularly frequent if primary pediatric headaches were migraine, although the headache classification often changes across time. Also, children with mild headaches at diagnosis are more likely to have remission than those with moderate or severe headaches, as the latter frequently continue to have moderate or severe headaches into adulthood.

Episodic TTH is usually associated with minimal to moderate discomfort and little disability, unless it evolves to the chronic form. In this case, the disability and use of medication escalate dramatically, leading to poorer outcomes and a higher risk for the patient to develop a MOH. At any rate, the prognosis for TTH tends to be even more favorable even in the more severe forms. Up to 45% of patients with frequent or chronic TTH go into remission within three years, with predictive factors for remission being older age and absence of chronic TTH at baseline.

CONCLUSION

Living with a headache disorder means facing many challenges beyond the headache itself. In this chapter we explored the hardships that headache patients must face as well as the damage inflicted by this condition to the entire human society as a whole. We also identified the many comorbidities and potential complications of headache and the long-term outcome for patients affected. The next chapter will focus on what impact these challenges and difficulties have on the families and friends of individuals with headaches.

7

Effects on Family and Friends

What makes it so difficult is that people think you are just having a regular headache. You just can't explain them to someone who doesn't have them.

—Kareem Abdul-Jabbar

Headaches and migraine aren't just misdiagnosed and poorly understood diseases. They are also misinterpreted conditions that are frequently underestimated by family and friends. Migraine in children is often dismissed as a tantrum, and even among adults, severe primary headache disorders are often seen as "just another headache." Few can understand the true pain and burden of living with migraine, cluster headache, or paroxysmal hemicrania, just to name a few. And fewer understand the challenges of taking care of someone affected by these curses.

While people living with a headache disorder must bear much of the true burden, they do not carry it all. This chapter will provide an ample overview of how this condition may affect family, friends, and other caregivers. While looking at this often overlooked facet of headache disorders, we will also provide many useful insights and advice on how to make the patient feel better beyond mere physical treatment. Ultimately, the goal of any caregiver and relative of headache sufferers is to help them share the burden and enjoy their lives to the fullest.

THE EFFECT OF CHRONIC HEADACHE ON FAMILY AND RELATIVES

Chronic illnesses are all associated with elevated family burden. In the United States, nearly one in four households includes someone with migraine, possibly even more than just one patient, since it tends to run in families. Anyone unfortunate enough to suffer from chronic or severe headache disorders understands very well how much these conditions not only cause physical suffering for the patient but also have a profound impact on the entire family. Unsurprisingly, illness severity is correlated with family impact, with more frequent and severe headaches having a much more substantial negative impact on other family members. People with chronic headaches often experience feelings of inadequacy, guilt, and sadness when they think about how their condition affects those they love. Opting out of family activities such as canceling vacations, missing social events, or having difficulty taking care of household and parenting responsibilities decreases the quality of the time spent with spouses and children for nearly half of all patients. Since headaches also impact career and educational accomplishments, financial achievements and economic stability are also jeopardized. Patients often think they would be better spouses and parents if they didn't have to live with such illnesses, and nearly one-third are worried about long-term financial security for themselves or their family because of their headaches.

Headaches cause relationships to be strained during and even between headache attacks. High levels of distress within relationships due to headache have been reported, especially when a couple's sexual life becomes affected as well. It is not infrequent for spouses or partners of patients with such conditions to have to take over parenting responsibilities such as disciplining, feeding, or carpooling and for children to be forced to take care of things that parents normally do for them (cooking, cleaning the house, etc.). More severe headaches have a much more significant emotional impact and burden on children who need to help their parents regularly. Two-thirds of children of people with migraine reportedly are made to keep quiet during attacks, and while one-third keep their distance, up to one-quarter have reported feeling confused, hostile, or afraid. A spouse or relative with a chronic headache can be perceived as even more demanding of the children because of the attacks. Approximately one-third of spouses of people with episodic migraine and nearly half of the spouses of those with chronic have reported avoiding the migraineur because of headache. Many sufferers perceive that their spouses and partners do not fully understand or believe the impact of their headaches, which further degrades their relationships. According to some studies, 5% of migraineurs interviewed admitted that migraine was the cause of their separation or divorce.

Headaches can damage relationships even when partners are not living together. Depending on the severity of the headache disorder, between 16% and 44% of subjects have claimed that their disorder caused relationship problems and/or contributed to preventing the relationship to bloom (by moving in together or getting married).

COMMON MYTHS ABOUT MIGRAINE AND SERIOUS HEADACHE DISORDERS

Along with being a very underdiagnosed condition, migraine is a frequently misunderstood disorder. The pain of living with migraine is often compounded by misconceptions that add insult to injury, making it even harder to live with. Other than perpetuating false information about the disease that contributes to aggravate it or prevent its correct diagnosis, these harmful myths can demoralize the patients and increase the burden they have to bear. Lack of support offered from family, friends, colleagues, and often even caregivers further contribute to the human cost of this invisible disease. In this section of the book, we want to put some of the most common myths about migraine to rest. Most of them can be applied to other serious headache disorders such as cluster headache, paroxysmal hemicrania, or hemicrania continua. Here's a short list:

1. *Migraine is just a headache.* This is by far the most common myth that surrounds many serious headache disorders. All migraineurs know very well that the most frequent answer they will get when telling other people about the condition is, "Yes, I also suffer from headaches." Hearing this repeated over and over constitutes a special form of pain on its own. Migraine is so much more than just a headache: it is a complex neurological disease, first and foremost. Its symptoms may last for up to several days and include serious neurological and autonomic features, and they are always severely disabling. A patient can't just "push through" a migraine attack and continue on with normal activities.

2. *If your headaches cause you so much suffering, why don't you go to the doctor?* It's not infrequent for doctors to underestimate a headache and prescribe inappropriate or ineffective medications to the patient. Migraines and other primary headaches are grossly underdiagnosed or misdiagnosed diseases. Some authors report that over 80% of migraines were misdiagnosed and managed as sinusitis, and less than half of patients had their condition diagnosed by a physician. And while 25% of sufferers could benefit from preventive treatment, only 12% of them actually receive it. Headache patients are often

discriminated against by health-care systems and are denied reimbursement for emergency room visits, hospitalizations, and sometimes even treatment.

3. **You suffer from migraine because you don't take enough meds.** In many cases, the truth is just the opposite. Too many medications (especially vaguely ineffective NSAIDs) can actually worsen the condition, making attacks become more frequent or intense. Too many medications may also cause rebound headaches and eventually lead to the dreaded medication-overuse headache (MOH).

4. **If there's no aura, then it's not a migraine/it's not a serious headache.** Roughly only one-third of all migraineurs experience aura, while everyone else may experience it once or twice in life or simply skip this stage altogether. Even people with aura may experience migraine without aura more than just occasionally. Many other of the most severe headache disorders are also not normally associated with symptoms of aura, such as trigeminal neuralgia, cluster headache, hemicrania continua, SUNCT/SUNA, and paroxysmal hemicrania.

5. **Actually, it's nothing serious; it's just stress, and you need to relax.** Although stress can be a contributing factor or even a trigger for some individuals, migraine isn't a psychological disorder or the product of some hysterical reaction that could be brushed off with a few words of dismissal. Migraine (or most other severe primary headaches) is a neurological disease that is linked with many altered physiological functions. Yoga and meditation may provide some bland relief and can probably help reduce the frequency of attacks, but they can't be listed as treatment for immensely painful conditions such as cluster headache—not even by a mile.

6. **I also had migraine, so I know what you're going through.** While this may be true to some extent, migraine includes a very broad range of features and symptoms that vary from person to person. Some symptoms are certainly common, but every subject affected by it experiences them in a different way. There are countless individual variations of migraine, each with their own unique set of symptoms, triggers, and response to treatment.

7. **You know what your migraine triggers are, and you just need to avoid them. If you still suffer from headache attacks, then it's your fault.** Although some of the triggers that are commonly associated with migraine and trigeminal autonomic cephalalgias (TACs) can be easily avoided (such as alcohol), not all of them are controllable. Good examples of uncontrollable headache triggers are weather changes or one's menstrual cycle. Even many of the controllable ones are sometimes not so easy to avoid. For example, monosodium glutamate (MSG), also

known as sodium glutamate, is a potent trigger, but it's commonly used as flavor to intensify the taste of many foods such as soy sauce, soups, and ramen. A migraineur may not know when glutamate is used to enhance the flavor of a dish or processed food, especially when eating at a restaurant or fast-food venue. Others, such as lack of sleep, stress, or negative life events, although technically controllable at least to some extent, may be hard to control in practice for many obvious reasons. Some may not be known by the headache patient since it's practically impossible to keep track of all the smells, odors, foods, and life circumstances that may trigger an attack. And even if all triggers are consistently avoided, sometimes an attack may occur no matter what, because that's what a headache does—like any other tragedy, it can strike when it is least expected.

8. ***Medications aren't effective; you should take this herbal remedy/supplement/essential oil instead.*** This myth is just the opposite of myth 2, but it is no less common. It is known that there are some herbal remedies that can provide some relief to people affected by headache disorders, such as St. John's wort (*Hypericum perforatum*), and that the strong smell of some perfumes may ease migraine pain (such as lavender oil). It is, however, true that these same remedies may actually worsen migraine in other people and that only specific medications such as triptans can provide relief during the stronger, more painful attacks. Not all supplements that prevent migraine are safe and effective, and—what's more important—they're not devoid of risks and side effects.

CARING FOR SOMEONE WITH MIGRAINE

Living with a severe headache disorder isn't easy, but caring for someone with such a condition is hardly a simple feat either. Having to see a patient writhing in pain or standing watch over the patient as the attack wanes can be a frightening experience, especially if the caring spouse, relative, or friend is not a professional caregiver. Yet for people living with migraine, cluster headache, or any other headache disorder, knowing that a loved one will have their back is extremely important. The health-care system can hardly, if ever, provide the kind of support and peace of mind that comes from the true dedication and love of a relative, spouse, or friend. Even small actions and thoughtful gestures can go a long way for those who must endure this torture for their entire life.

Understanding what affected individuals are experiencing is the first step to being able to aid loved ones, provide proper support and care, and ultimately help them suffer less, live better, and get more control over the disorder. For example, what's comforting during a certain phase of a migraine can be irritating or disturbing when the pain reaches its peak. Some foods, perfumes, sounds, or even everyday chores, such as making the bed, can become dreadful triggers for a migraineur, and knowing how to avoid them is a critical component of effective prevention. Being supportive of individuals with a severe headache requires respecting their need to rest, avoid interactions, and be protected from stimuli (lights, sounds, odors, etc.). Knowing that home is a safe haven where they can endure the attack with minimum pain is crucial for patients' physical and mental health.

One of the most important things to do is to never underestimate and understate the suffering associated with a major headache. Even when a patient is determined or stubborn enough to soldier through an attack, this does not mean that the symptoms the patient is enduring aren't exhausting. Severe headache disorders are invisible diseases, and it's not infrequent for them to be disregarded as the simplest headache that all experience at least once during their lives. According to some studies, nearly three-quarters of friends or relatives of people with migraine do not believe that the headache attacks are as severe as the patients report. However, few things are more heart-wrenching for headache patients than to feel that their loved ones do not believe them when they say they are in pain. This, in turn, also means that caregivers should always back care recipients up when another party falls prey to the most common misconceptions about headache disorders. Stepping in and having their back—for example, when a boss is expecting them to deliver at work or when someone minimizes the pain they're facing—can make a big difference.

Although headache disorders will unavoidably cause some plans to get canceled and some family events to get missed, knowing how not to make the patients feel guilty about that or bad about what they can't do is important for their psychological well-being. Sometimes, the easier thing to do is to find fun activities that can be done together that won't trigger a headache, such as watching a movie instead of going to a rock concert. After all, one should always remember that people with headaches just want a normal life as anyone else, and they're doing all they can to live life to the fullest despite all the hurt. And for them, nothing is more important than knowing that the people they love are able to see through their condition and care about them.

THE UNIQUE CHALLENGES POSED BY HEADACHE AND MIGRAINE IN CHILDREN

Migraine in children arguably is the most misunderstood and under-recognized form of headache. When kids claim to have a headache, it is easy to imagine they are just throwing a tantrum to avoid going to school. But headaches in children can be a frequent and highly disabling neurological disorder. Migraine actually is the most common cause of acute recurrent headaches in children and adolescents and one of the top five diseases of childhood. About 10% of school-age children suffer from migraine, and up to 28% of adolescents between 15 and 19 years of age are affected by it. Half of all migraine sufferers experienced their first attack before the age of 12, but the condition has been reported in infants as young as 18 months. It is probably even more prevalent than we think, as more recent studies have pointed out how infant colic can be associated with childhood migraine and may even be an early form of migraine. It is possible that pediatric patients with cyclic syndromes such as abdominal migraine, benign paroxysmal vertigo, cyclic vomiting syndrome, and benign paroxysmal torticollis either already have migraine or are prone to eventually develop it.

Migraine has been found to account for up to 18% of patients in the pediatric emergency room. Despite this, serious headaches in children and adolescents are frequently ignored by parents, teachers, and primary-care providers as well, resulting in lost school days and impaired social interactions. The negative impact of migraines on a child's overall quality of life is so severe that it has been compared to that of pediatric cancer, heart disease, and rheumatic disease. Kids and teens with headaches may develop anticipatory anxiety as they worry that the next attack will disrupt their lives, and their chance of being absent from school is two times higher than those who don't suffer from these conditions.

The familial risk of migraine has been established by substantial evidence, with a 50% chance for children to inherit it if they have one parent with migraine and a 75% chance if both parents have migraine. This means that children with migraine must often live in households where other family members share their burden, generating an even more stressful environment to live in. Stress always negatively impacts a migraineur's health, but children's psychoemotional stability can be affected even more because of their heavy dependence on their caregivers. Preexisting problems with family communication can lead to increased problems with pain management and worse health outcomes. Increased stressors on and from family are often positively correlated with higher levels of disability during childhood as well as adulthood, contributing to an overall less favorable prognosis. Unlike in adults, the incidence of migraine is higher in males than in females before puberty. However, the number changes by the time they turn 17, with as many as 8% of boys and 23% of girls having experienced a migraine.

Although no less disabling, symptoms of migraine in kids and teens can be different from those typically found in adults, accounting, at least in part, for the high number of misdiagnosed or undiagnosed cases. Pain can be frontal rather than temporal or occipital, and bilateral rather than unilateral, although in some cases, the presentation is the same as in adults. Focal pain is generally consistent with migraine, whereas a more diffuse description of pain may be consistent with tension-type headaches (TTHs). Gastrointestinal symptoms such as nausea, abdominal pain, and vomiting tend to be more prominent in children. Diagnosis is also difficult in young children, as the condition is defined by subjective symptoms that can't be properly described. Concepts that are harder to grasp and describe such as photophobia and phonophobia must be inferred by the parents on the basis of the child's actions. Other less evident symptoms include dizziness, sleep disturbances, anxiety, depression, difficulty concentrating, and fatigue and can become chronic or present even between episodes. Headache attacks also tend to be shorter in duration, usually lasting between 2 and 72 hours. Since the diagnosis of migraine in children and adolescents usually requires being established through a headache history, involving the parents and helping them recognize the disease is especially important.

Pediatric treatment of migraine is quite similar as in adulthood, since children are often managed as "little adults" and their pharmacological treatment is titrated accordingly. The same abortive and preventive medications are prescribed at lower doses since once a treatment is deemed effective in adults, it is typically used in the pediatric population as well. However, no rigorous scientific assessment is usually made prior to implementation in patients under the age of 18, so, although common, this approach may not reflect best practice. In fact, some recent trials showed how treatment with certain drugs, such as amitriptyline or topiramate, are not as effective in pediatric populations as in adults and are associated with significantly more adverse events. Pharmacological therapies that have been studied rigorously for use in pediatric patients include ibuprofen, acetaminophen, almotriptan, rizatriptan, and the nasal spray forms of sumatriptan and zolmitriptan. They are all safe and effective in controlling migraine and TTH but must be used with caution to avoid the development of a MOH. Lifestyle and dietary recommendations, on the other hand, can be more effective in children than in adults, possibly because of the higher adherence to these recommendations. Patient education can also significantly enhance all health outcomes, such as weight loss in obese children, bringing many additional benefits beyond improvement of headaches only.

Early recognition of migraine is critical to promptly establish a treatment plan and the implementation of lifestyle changes that could improve the child's quality of life. Migraine and the other serious headaches are not the benign, self-limited disorders they were previously thought to be. People who experience migraine episodes during childhood often continue to suffer them into adulthood. Therefore, altering the disease progression as early as possible is no less important when migraines frequently have their onset during early to mid-adolescence. In other words, understanding the trajectory of severe headaches from childhood to adulthood is a fundamental step in establishing an efficient, lifetime approach to patient care.

CONCLUSION

Despite their tremendous impact on patients' lives and society as a whole, major headache disorders are still shrouded in myth and misinformation, and it's hard to tell whether misdiagnosis and mistreatment are a cause or a consequence of such popular misperceptions. For centuries, the medical community and society as a whole blamed headaches on their sufferers, so it comes as no surprise how frequently these disorders are underestimated by relatives and even caregivers. This chapter's purpose was to arm those living with headache patients with the real facts and mechanics of these complex disorders to improve the quality of life of those affected. In the next chapter, we will see how prevention is critical in reducing the burden of headaches by minimizing their severity and frequency, as well as what hygienic countermeasures may be utilized to achieve optimal management of these challenging diseases.

8

Prevention

The sooner you can attack the headache, the better. Whether you're an actress or you're a teacher or you're the postman, you have a job to do ... and you can't be shut down for two days because of a migraine.

—Jennie Garth

Many headaches are nothing but a minor ailment that goes away on its own after a few hours. However, a headache disorder is a serious condition that profoundly impacts the lives of the patients affected. People dealing with chronic or recurring headaches are often worried that their disease is not taken seriously, and the very fact that a doctor takes their concerns seriously is often enough to have a therapeutic effect. Patient reassurance is a critical step in the therapeutic process, and a thorough examination of all trigger factors can have many beneficial effects on overall health outcomes. When it comes to headaches, knowledge is power. The more knowledge patients have about their disorder, the better they can avoid triggers, and the lower the risk of abusing abortive medications that could worsen the headache or lead to medication-overuse headache (MOH).

Information about the nature of the disease and its physiological mechanisms has proven to make prognosis more favorable in the long run. Prevention is nowadays considered a staple of any and all headache therapies and is often the preferred therapeutic approach to achieve optimal management of the disorder. This chapter will explore headache prevention and hygiene and how lifestyle changes or appropriate preventive approaches are able to lesser the burden of headache.

NUTRACEUTICALS AND DIETARY SUPPLEMENTS

For many patients with a primary headache disorder who need long-term prescription treatments to manage their disease, current pharmacologic therapies can eventually cause a range of issues and side effects. People with migraines or severe headaches use complementary and alternative medicine more often than those without, because conventional treatments are frequently perceived as ineffective or too costly. In particular, dietary supplements and nutraceuticals can provide medicinal effects and some pain relief that are sometimes quite effective and more tolerable than conventional treatment. More often than not, vitamins, minerals, and herbal remedies are perceived as less toxic than prescription medication, although this may not necessarily be the case. Currently, the evidence for some nutraceuticals is promising, but lack of sufficiently large, rigorous clinical studies and inconsistent results leads to a widespread skepticism among the medical community. Although this kind of nonpharmacological or quasi-pharmacological therapy is still used and appreciated by many, international guidelines do not always agree on their safety and effectiveness, and recommendations are ultimately conflicting.

The most commonly used nutraceuticals that have shown some evidence in migraine prevention are magnesium, supplements for mitochondrial dysfunction (vitamin B_2, coenzyme Q10, and alpha-lipoic acid), and preventive herbal remedies (butterbur root extract and feverfew).

Magnesium

Magnesium is an essential element that is involved in neurotransmission and other important physiological processes. Previous studies have highlighted a possible role of this mineral in migraine pathogenesis. Magnesium deficiency has been associated with some specific pathogenetic mechanisms of migraine, such as cortical spreading depression, and the release of some neurotransmitters or pain mediators such as substance P, as well as other nonspecific pathogenetic mechanisms that are common in other headache disorders, including platelet aggregation and vasoconstriction. In addition, ionized magnesium plays a critical role in inhibiting glutamate expression through NMDA receptor binding. However, since magnesium levels in soft tissues cannot be reliably measured, the association between magnesium deficiency and severe headache still remains hypothetical. Both oral and intravenous supplementation of magnesium has been tested, but results are somehow inconsistent. Evidence suggesting that magnesium may constitute an effective preventive treatment for migraine patients is still limited, and it is important to remember that higher doses of this mineral can become toxic (hypermagnesemia).

Supplements for Mitochondrial Dysfunction

An impairment in mitochondrial oxygen metabolism is another one of the potential dysfunctions suggested as a pathogenic mechanism for migraine and other headaches. A reduction in oxygen levels could lower the threshold for headache attacks, and an impairing of the mitochondrial phosphorylation potential has been found in migraine patients between attacks. Supplements that enhance mitochondrial function should, therefore, ameliorate the symptoms of migraineurs, and possibly reduce the frequency of attacks by rising their threshold. The most commonly used supplements for mitochondrial dysfunction include vitamin B_2 (riboflavin), coenzyme Q10 (CoQ10), and alpha-lipoic acid.

Vitamin B_2 (Riboflavin)

Vitamin B_2 is a component of flavin mononucleotide and flavin adenine dinucleotide. These two important coenzymes are cofactors in the electron transport chain of the Krebs cycle and are required for several energy-related cellular functions. Riboflavin plays a central role in improving membrane stability and maintaining healthy cellular functions; therefore, it may be beneficial in migraine prophylaxis. To date, the studies that have assessed the efficacy of riboflavin in migraine have shown somewhat conflicting results. One possible explanation for these differences is that ethnic variations in mitochondrial DNA may influence the response to riboflavin, as has been suggested by recent pharmacogenetic studies. On the other hand, a small study postulated that riboflavin and beta blockers could act synergistically on two distinct aspects of migraine pathophysiology, explaining why vitamin B_2 could be more effective in patients who are taking concomitant preventive treatments. In any case, current evidence seems to be sufficient to recommend the use of riboflavin as a well-tolerated, low-risk preventive treatment for adults with migraine.

Coenzyme Q10 (CoQ10)

Like riboflavin, coenzyme Q10 (CoQ10) is an enzyme cofactor involved in the mitochondrial electron transport chain and energy metabolism. Its usefulness in headache prevention has been hypothesized because of its role in aerobic cellular respiration and for its marked antioxidant properties. CoQ10 is well tolerated by most patients, and it doesn't have side effects other than mild ones such as stomach troubles or nausea. However, it could be contraindicated during concomitant therapy with blood thinners, and doses higher than 300 milligrams can show signs of liver toxicity. Although to this day evidence about the effectiveness of CoQ10 still remains insufficient, some studies identified it as a promisingly effective substance in the prophylaxis of migraine, especially in the pediatric population.

Alpha-lipoic acid

Alpha-lipoic acid or 6,8-thioctic acid is an endogenous fatty acid that can be found in many foods such as yeast extract, broccoli, spinach, and organ meats (e.g., kidney or heart). It functions as an important cofactor for various mitochondrial enzymes, augmenting their oxygen metabolism and production of adenosine triphosphate. Alpha-lipoic acid could also act by lowering the insulin resistance that may occur in some migraineurs, and it is known for its neuroprotective and anti-inflammatory effects. The levels of this fatty acid have also been found to remain low in migraine patients. As for other nutraceutical supplements, the studies that suggest the benefits of alpha-lipoic acid in migraine prophylaxis are still insufficient.

Preventive Herbal Remedies

In chapter 5, we already mentioned some herbs and phytotherapic preparations as potential agents to treat migraine. However, we mostly focused on those remedies that could stop a headache in its tracks (abortive agents) rather than those herbal extracts that could show some efficacy in prophylaxis. The two herbs that show the most promise as preventives are butterbur and feverfew.

Butterbur root (Petasites hybridus)

One of the herbal extracts that have shown much promise in recent years is butterbur root (*Petasites hybridus*). The name of this perennial shrub found in Europe and Asia derives from the leaves of the plant, which were used in the past to wrap butter because of their size. Butterbur extract has a long history as a natural remedy for fever, pain, spasms, and wound healing. The mechanism of action of the sesquiterpenes, such as petasin and isopetasin, found in the plant is not fully understood yet. Apparently, active compounds known as petasites act by regulating calcium channels and inhibiting the biosynthesis of peptide leukotriene, thus influencing the inflammatory cascade associated with migraine. It is interesting to note how one of the most important pharmaceutical compounds used in the prophylaxis of cluster headache is the calcium channel blocker verapamil. The plant itself is, however, somewhat dangerous to use, since it also contains pyrrolizidine alkaloids, which are hepatotoxic and carcinogenic. However, in commercially available preparations, these substances are removed, so all products certified and labeled as "PA-free" should be safe for human use. In contrast to other nutraceuticals, most studies about butterbur extracts agree about its effectiveness in decreasing the frequency of migraine attacks. However, it cannot currently be recommended as a preventive treatment due to the safety concerns noted above.

Feverfew (Tanacetum parthenium)

Feverfew (*Tanacetum parthenium*) is a medicinal herb that was consistently employed across human history in the treatment of a broad range of different ailments such as headache, fevers, infertility, toothaches, and arthritis. Originally native to the Balkan Mountains, it now grows throughout Europe, North America, and South America. Its antiheadache action is probably due to the ability of the parthenolides found in the leaves to inhibit platelet aggregation and to the release of serotonin from platelets and white blood cells. An additional anti-inflammatory action, through the inhibition of prostaglandin synthesis and phospholipase A, could also help in headache prophylaxis.

Tolerability and safety of feverfew seem good, with most reported side effects being mild: gastrointestinal disturbances, mouth ulcers, and joint aches. More serious adverse reactions are reported in patients with allergies and in pregnant women; it is not recommended for the latter as it may cause uterine contractions resulting in miscarriage or preterm labor. At any rate, current studies are few in number and inconsistent, and they have failed to provide convincing evidence on the effectiveness of this herb in migraine prophylaxis. Inconsistencies in results may, however, originate from the wide variations in the strength of the leaves' parthenolides and the differences in the stability of herbal extract preparations, so more research is ultimately needed.

VITAMIN D

Vitamin D is a group of fat-soluble vitamins, the most important of which in humans are vitamin D_2 (also known as ergocalciferol) and vitamin D_3 (cholecalciferol). Naturally present in a small number of foods, vitamin D is normally produced endogenously through exposure to direct sunlight rays. Ultraviolet (UV) irradiation of the skin triggers vitamin D synthesis and metabolism. The final product of this metabolism is calcitriol, the biologically active form of vitamin D, which is known to be central in many physiological processes such as calcium metabolism, bone growth and remodeling, modulation of inflammation, immune function, and glucose metabolism.

According to a recent literature review, a growing number of published studies show a link between low serum vitamin D levels and headaches, especially for migraine and cluster headache. The current literature seemingly indicates that vitamin D may be beneficial in some headache patients, at least in those with confirmed deficiency of this substance. It must, however, be noted that vitamin D deficiency is an emerging global health problem that affects up to 30%–80% of children and adults worldwide. Epidemiologic data on headache show a higher prevalence with increasing latitude (e.g., where exposure to UV rays is decreased), an increased frequency of headaches in autumn and winter, and a decreased number of attacks during the summer that match the serum vitamin D levels seasonal variations.

The mechanism through which vitamin D may reduce frequency and severity of headaches is still unknown. Vitamin D receptors are found in many regions of the brain, so it is likely that calcitriol has specific functions in regulating brain development, as a neuroprotective agent, and in contributing to the vascular health of the brain. Vitamin D and its metabolites can influence several neurotransmitters known to be connected with the pathogenesis of migraine, including serotonin, dopamine, and nitric oxide. Some studies pointed out how deficiency increases the risk of neurological diseases, such as stroke and dementia, as well as pain disorders, such as arthritis and muscle pain. The anti-inflammatory properties of vitamin D may also be central in modulating or downregulating the inflammatory substances produced during headache attacks that activate the trigeminovascular system.

Vitamin D supplementation appears to be a safe form of preventive headache treatment even at high dose (5,000–10,000 IU per day or 50,000 IU per week), with no major adverse events reported. While evidence to recommend vitamin D supplementation to every patient with a headache is still not enough, some authors claim that this substance may be beneficial to reduce the frequency of headaches at least in those with a confirmed reduction in serum levels.

THE EFFECTS OF STRESS

Stress or, even worse, anxiety can be either a direct cause or a factor in triggering headaches. Emotional stress, anxiety, shock, tension, unhappiness, and depression can directly cause tension headaches and migraine attacks. According to the American Headache Society, roughly four out of five patients affected by migraines report stress as a trigger, and there is evidence that stress can also contribute to migraine chronification. Many unhealthy habits associated with stress, such as skipping meals, alcohol use, smoking, or losing sleep, may also cause tension headache, migraine, or other primary headache attacks. Studies have found a link between migraine headaches and stress, as the pain of the headache itself generates more stress, creating a vicious cycle. The interaction between stress and migraine may result from biochemical changes related to the physiological stress response, such as the release of corticotrophin-releasing hormone, although individual variations in personal response to stressors, rather than stressors themselves, represent a major factor.

Literature has amply documented the pervasive and destructive impact of headaches on patients' life and how these insidious diseases can catch their victims in a vicious cycle of never-ending stress. Negative interpersonal situations and circumstances arising from a primary headache condition, such as shame or embarrassment related to migraine attacks or lifestyle limitations, can have a tremendously affective and psychological impact. Stress resulting from headaches can negatively impact social and professional areas, generate negative social interactions, and modify the disposition of others. This contributes to reducing the overall quality of life of headache patients, their ability to obtain adequate care, and their psychological experience of the condition, and thus it increases their stress level more and more.

Especially if this stress is experienced since childhood or early adolescence, it may contribute to make the individual's psychological balance frailer and less prone to cope with negative events. As the icing on a cake made of pain, high levels of stress are known to lead to a higher prevalence of psychological disorders such as depression and anxiety, which are associated with a more negative prognosis for headache. To add insult to injury, if people with headache are labeled as "sensitive" by others because of their personality or psychological background, chances that their attacks are brushed off as a somatization of their inability to cope with stress. As we already explained in chapter 7, few things can hurt the feelings of migraineurs or clusterheads more than not being believed about the seriousness of their condition. Hence, while stress could be considered a cause of migraines due to its interpersonal impact, at the same time, it shouldn't be, as it is only part of a particularly callous chain of circumstances that many headache patients must frequently face.

On top of all that, when a patient's body grows accustomed to constant stress, a sudden reduction in stress levels may trigger a headache episode resulting in a so-called weekend headache or letdown migraine. This form of "Sunday syndrome" is very common in those patients who keep their headaches under control during the week while they perform very stressful activities (in the workplace, at school, while caring for children, etc.). As soon as the week is over, these poor souls can't even enjoy their weekend, as they spend most of it in bed with a breakthrough attack. Needless to say, this disruption in weekend plans or family activities will lead to further stress, preventing the victim from resting and taking a break before another stressful week begins. Although the causes of these unusual "holiday headaches" still remain a mystery, some authors have theorized that higher stress levels on weekdays can lead the body to increase its production of glucocorticoids as an adaptive response. The sudden drop in glucocorticoid levels may cause the headache, through a mechanism similar to what happens when patients are treated with steroids. It has also been suggested that inconsistent sleeping patterns on weekdays followed by oversleeping during the weekend may also act as a trigger, as can caffeine withdrawal if a person normally consumes large amounts of caffeine-containing substances during the week.

Ultimately, the right adaptive coping strategies and healthy lifestyle choices can go a long way toward protecting patients from the worst presentations of a primary headache disorder. Since the individual's responses to stressors seem to be more important than the stressors themselves in initiating the headache episodes, learning how to effectively manage and cope with stress has a greater potential for reducing the impact of stress than trying to avoid stressors altogether. Relaxation techniques, physical exercise, and consistent sleep schedules can all have a beneficial effect that should not be underestimated. For many patients, having more control over their condition and symptoms, as well as their lives as a whole, can help reduce stress and, in turn, reduce the frequency and sometimes even the severity of the attacks. However, despite the importance of reducing stress levels, this alone can never fully prevent attacks from occurring, with the exception of some less severe cases of tension-type headache (TTH).

MANAGEMENT AND PROPHYLAXIS

Prevention and prophylactic strategies are vital to stop the transformation of most headache disorders from episodic into chronic. It is a known fact that many headaches such as migraine, TTH, and cluster headache tend to worsen over time when they're not adequately managed. Although the pathogenetic mechanisms beyond this transformation are still unclear, it is possible that frequent central sensitization may tend to perpetuate the headache. Proper treatment must be administered in the right amount, because while an ignored disease may grow out of control, too much of a treatment can also be an issue, with MOHs being a constant threat to headache patients.

This introduced the paradigm of early intervention, an approach where treatment is administered early in the attack while the headache is still mild. Optimal treatment should be achieved by finely tuning therapy for each patient. The goal is to know the migraine's pattern as well as possible, learn what triggers it, and take the minimum number of drugs possible only during the patient's own window of vulnerability. Early treatment is important but may encourage more frequent use of abortive medications such as triptans or NSAIDs when beginning attacks have not yet evolved into full-blown headaches. Patients, scared by the symptoms of a painful and disabling attack, may start using abortive medications as prophylactic ones and become prone to the consequences of overuse.

When appropriate management of acute headaches cannot be achieved, patients should be evaluated for initiation of preventive therapy. The goal of prophylactic therapy is to improve patients' quality of life by reducing migraine frequency, severity, and duration and by increasing the responsiveness of acute migraines to treatment. Preventive therapies are recommended in patients with chronic, severe, or frequent headaches and in patients who do not tolerate or fail to respond to abortive treatment. The drugs used for the prophylaxis of headaches pertain to many different categories, ranging from beta blockers to calcium channel blockers, tricyclic antidepressants, and anticonvulsants. They are either specifically approved for the prevention of trigeminal autonomic cephalalgias (TACs), migraine, and the other headache disorders, or they have class A evidence supporting their use. However, patients' adherence to treatment and compliance are frequently poor, due to the drugs' side effects and somewhat modest efficacy. Prophylactic treatment is, in fact, not curative, and most patients will still need abortive medications for acute attacks. Choosing the right agent that balances efficacy, side effects, contraindications, and cost is thus critical to maximize adherence to treatment.

LIFESTYLE, DIET, AND THE IMPORTANCE OF THE MIGRAINE DIARY

Lifestyle and environment are known to trigger migraines and TACs. We have already discussed how some foods and substances, weather changes, altitude changes, altered sleep habits, and stress can be important triggers that most headache sufferers painfully learn to avoid. Once these conditions are encountered, the cascade of events leading to a full-blown attack within a couple of hours or days will ensue. A vicious cycle may develop: the more frequently the neurovascular pathways involved in primary headaches are stimulated, the worse the inflammation becomes, lowering the threshold to flare a headache every time the patient faces one of such triggers. In other words, knowing what one can and what one cannot do is critical to minimize the risk of facing a devastating attack that will just make things even worse in the long term.

Eating and living healthy can decrease the number of attacks by reducing overall inflammation. In a less inflamed organism, migrainous stimulation requires reaching a higher threshold before an attack is fired. But while a healthy lifestyle and diet are important, knowing exactly what triggers a headache attack in each patient is a challenge that only patients themselves can (and should) overcome. Attacks may flare some days after triggers occur, and these triggers may change over the course of life, making it hard to determine them with sufficient precision. In particular, many common foods such as cheese or wine may contain chemicals, such as tyramine, that are known migraine triggers. And foods that are harmless in their natural forms may end up containing triggers such as MSG, among other preservatives and flavorings, when they are processed. When migraine-triggering foods are identified, restricting their intake can be an effective and reliable preventive intervention. Therefore, it is important for the patients to be able to track all the changes in their health to be able to spot even the most unsuspecting dietary triggers.

To a different degree and for different reasons, lifestyle can strongly affect TTH. Many patients who suffer from the more severe forms of this condition may find great relief by simply changing some of their habits, since this headache may be caused by a wrong walking posture, nocturnal bruxism (involuntary teeth grinding or jaw clenching), improper seating, and muscle contractions. Even simple, everyday changes such as changing a chair, a pillow, or a pair of shoes can effectively prevent TTHs or even intervene at the root of the issue.

Although primary headaches are often described or perceived as unpredictable, up to 70% of migraine patients have prodromal warning symptoms that may be identified with a sufficient degree of self-awareness. Several national and international headache organizations recommend that patients keep a diary to track the characteristics of their headaches. Widely known as the "migraine diary," this diary can prove to be highly beneficial in many other headaches such as TTHs and TACs. Inside the migraine diary, the patient will keep track of the frequency, duration, and severity of the headaches over time and maintain a record of all medications taken and their response (or lack thereof). Keeping detailed records of headache episodes can help in providing additional insight about triggers and how to avoid them and can be used to build a headache history, for the benefit of the diagnosis process and for management purposes. Important details such as when the headaches start, how often they occur, where the pain is, and whether other symptoms are present can be instrumental in structuring a proper differential diagnosis. The diary can help doctors and patients identify headache patterns, determine which medication is more effective, spot potentially undiscovered triggers, titrate dosage to the minimum required, reduce the risk of MOH, and improve adherence to therapy and compliance. It is also helpful from a more holistic point of view, since by keeping track of everyday information such as daily hours of sleep, skipped meals, physical exercise, and social and work activities, it can contribute to a healthier lifestyle. Filling a diary also promotes a deeper understanding of the disease, making the patient more self-aware and therefore proactive in avoiding triggers and stressors which may contribute to poorer health outcomes.

In modern times, internet-based headache diaries and smartphone apps have been implemented to further expand the concept of migraine diary. Digital diaries (also known as electronic diaries or e-diaries) are often preferred to physical ones due to their simplicity and immediateness. They can operate on virtually any device that can connect to the internet and allow patients to keep track of the characteristics of their headaches (duration, severity, aura, etc.), triggers (stress, lack of sleep, food, etc.), medications taken, and the medications' effectiveness and can also facilitate communication with health-care providers. Keeping electronic diaries have proved to be valuable for patients in that, by doing so, they have a much easier time identifying their triggers and adhering to therapy. They are powerful tools for health-care providers as well. Specialists can easily follow the patient's progress between visits, measure treatment compliance, and have access to detailed reports and insights that remove many of the traditional doctor-patient barriers. E-diaries are extremely useful for data collection purposes and to recruit and retain geographically diverse populations who have not previously participated in research studies and clinical trials.

CONCLUSION

This chapter discussed the importance of prevention and prophylaxis in tackling the apparently unsurmountable challenge of living with a serious headache. We explored some of the less visible factors that contribute to make headaches worse and/or more frequent and how headaches might be avoided or prevented. We highlighted the most effective strategies to pre-vent and overall ameliorate the health outcomes and quality of life of a patient affected by a headache disorder.

In the next chapter, we will discuss the most controversial aspects of headache treatment and management as well as some of the nastiest social implications of living with this burden.

9

Issues and Controversies

If the headache would only precede the intoxication, alcoholism would be a virtue.

—Samuel Butler

This chapter will focus on the most important controversies or debates related to headache, on both the medical and sociocultural levels. Migraine and the other headache disorders are underestimated and undertreated conditions, and people affected must frequently face stigma due to prejudice as well as substantial barriers to effective care. We will also discuss about some of the controversial approaches to treatment that involve the use of illegal substances, as well as the most heated medical debates about the pathogenesis of the disease.

BARRIERS TO EFFECTIVE CARE

Headache disorders are among the most prevalent disorders of humankind, yet worldwide neglect of these conditions is appalling. Despite representing a ubiquitous and highly prevalent public health problem associated with enormous financial costs to society and personal burden, headache disorders are universally underrecognized, underdiagnosed, and undertreated.

Although most patients troubled or disabled by headaches are largely treatable, there is substantial evidence that a huge percentage of them do not receive effective health care. For example, in the United States and the United Kingdom, only half of those identified with migraine were seen by a doctor for headache-related reasons in the previous year, and only two-thirds were correctly diagnosed. Most had no access to prescription drugs and had to rely on over-the-counter medications, exposing themselves to a significant risk of developing medication-overuse headache (MOH). And in resource-poor countries, the situation is generally even worse than in the most developed countries of the world.

The barriers responsible for reduced access to effective care range from clinical to social, political, and economic ones, but general lack of awareness and limited access to resources represent critical issues virtually everywhere. They occur on various levels. Mostly, as we already said, a lot of people with a headache do not consult doctors. When they do, they do not receive the correct diagnosis. And even if they receive the correct diagnosis, many do not receive the right treatment for their condition.

Clinical Barriers

Better professional education for specialists who treat headache disorders is seen as one of the key issues impeding appropriate management of these conditions. Only slightly more than half of the specialists worldwide use the *ICHD* (in any of its present or past iterations) during the diagnosis process, especially in Africa, Southeast Asia, and the eastern Mediterranean. On the other hand, if people with headache do not consult doctors for social or cultural reasons, headache management guidelines for doctors become less important, while guidelines for other health-care providers (such as nurses or clinical officers) become much more relevant. In any case, very little is done to encourage proper understanding of the diseases, with just 4 hours being committed to headache disorders in formal undergraduate medical training and 10 hours in specialist training.

Professional organizations for headache disorders are fundamental in improving the understanding of the disease. They arrange conferences, raise awareness of headache-related issues, and are involved in setting guidelines in the management of headache disorders. However, one-third of the world's countries have no professional organization, and the percentage is even lower in low-income countries alone (16%). Also, very few of them participate in the construction of postgraduate or undergraduate training curricula (20% and 10%, respectively).

There's much room for improvement of headache care at the education level, especially in less-developed countries. Greater investment in health care to diagnose and treat headache more effectively is necessary through well-organized health services supported by education. In turn, this investment would certainly be associated with important monetary savings due to the enormous indirect costs of these disorders.

Political and Economic Barriers

Many governments fail to acknowledge the substantial burden of headache on society and the amount of money and resources that could be saved if appropriate measures to manage these disorders were taken. Some headache disorders such as cluster headache, trigeminal autonomic cephalalgias (TACs) and migraine contribute much more substantially to public ill-health than other, more common ones, such as tension-type headache (TTH), that do not necessarily require medical intervention to be treated. However, a proper assessment of the actual impact of headache is currently not possible since very few countries have run sufficient population-based studies from which national-level data could be derived. Detailed comparisons of headache disorders with other common and disabling ones are the foundation upon which adequate health-care provision and informed public health policies must be built.

In countries where resources to manage headaches are scant, patients' access to care and effective treatments is much more limited. Similarly, in less-developed countries where health-care systems in general must struggle with lack of funding, finding adequate treatment for headache disorders may be impossible, since the few resources available are concentrated on more urgent issues (such as infective diseases). However, even in more-developed countries, patients seeking treatment must face many economic barriers. In particular, health insurance status can be an important predictor of consulting, and the high cost of some medications or long-term prophylactic therapy could constitute a challenge for people in the lower-income bracket.

Cultural and Social Barriers

Lack of awareness and understanding of headaches is present in the general public as well. As we already discussed in previous chapters, headache disorders are often trivialized since they are not contagious, are ubiquitous, and are rarely (if ever) deadly. Minimization of more severe headache disorders leads to a generalized stigma toward people affected by them, who are often seen as idlers who look for an excuse to avoid responsibility. A direct consequence is that people who may otherwise benefit from treatment may avoid seeking help from doctors, fearing stigma, reprisal, and an emotional burden. This issue is even more accentuated in those societies that are especially focused on production; one example is Japan, where migraine and rates of consultation by those with migraine were found to be noticeably low. General dismissal of migraine and more severe headaches may also be one of the reasons why women have been far more likely to be diagnosed than men have been, as current data suggest that gender bias in diagnosis constitutes another important barrier for men.

At any rate, lack of awareness about the more serious headache diseases, which are often confused with milder ones such as episodic TTH, exists even among people who are directly affected by them. It's not infrequent for people with migraine or cluster headache to be unaware that their conditions require special medical care, leading to abuse of self-treatment medications and consequently MOH. Needless to say, the situation is even worse in less-developed countries. In some regions, tradition or religious beliefs may prevent some people from looking for appropriate care. At the same time, clinging to alternative or complementary therapies deeply rooted in religion, esotericism, pseudoscience, or plain quackery may be systematically preferred to effective treatment in some cultures.

The Stigma Associated with Migraine

Stigma is a recognized social construct that describes a characteristic, trait, or diagnosis that is used to damage the reputation of an individual and cause their loss of status; it is associated with discrimination and prejudice. Stigmatization spoils the identity of the affected individual and occurs with some neurological or psychiatric diseases such as epilepsy, depression, psychosis, and migraine for a broad range of social and historical reasons. The effects of stigmatization are known to disrupt social relationships and careers and to further worsen the quality of life of individuals stigmatized, thus negatively impacting the health outcomes of such patients. When it occurs, individuals experience discrimination, loss of employment, and subjective stressful experiences that can damage their health. Eventually, stigma becomes internalized and incorporated into the individuals' own identity and can lead to negative reactions in anticipation of how other people may perceive them, further reinforcing its overall impact.

Migraine patients started to be looked down upon starting in the late eighteenth century, when they were depicted as privileged, self-absorbed individuals who took advantage of their headaches as an excuse for shirking social duties and avoiding social responsibilities. In the nineteenth century, however, this view took a steep turn when migraine started to be described as a weakness of women in the lower socioeconomic classes. Migraine itself was seen as a psychological defect or hysteria resulting from the excitable female brain. Even physicians who took care of patients affected by chronic or recurrent headaches were ridiculed as wacky, incompetent practitioners who encouraged their patients' neurotic tendencies. Eventually, this negative, gender-stereotyped view of the person with a migraine became an established social construct, with migraine patients being perceived as hysterical, overemotional, and negatively feminized individuals. It is very possible that since this stigma impacts men in a much more severe way than it does women, it could be one of the reasons why headache disorders are more frequently underdiagnosed and undertreated in male patients.

Although it occurs in migraine at least as much as in those with epilepsy or panic disorder, stigma is an underrecognized feature of headache disorders with important consequences in disrupting patients' social, family, and working life. Due to the emotional burden it adds, stigma can influence both the patient's willingness to seek treatment and health outcomes in general. Like any other highly stressful circumstance, stigma can make headache attacks become more frequent or severe, especially in chronic patients. Destigmatization is, therefore, necessary and must take place at the level of both patients and health-care providers since stigma is a serious public health problem that ultimately affects the chances for patients to receive effective treatment.

THE EFFECTS OF PSYCHEDELICS AND PSYCHOTROPICS ON CLUSTER HEADACHE AND MIGRAINE

The history of the use of psychedelic or psychotropic substances to treat cluster headache and migraine is deeply intertwined with the history of the early World Wide Web. In late 1998, a man posted a message on an internet bulletin board claiming one of his cluster cycles was prevented by taking the hallucinogen lysergic acid diethylamide (LSD). He kept experimenting with other indole-ring hallucinogens, posting his successful results on the board. Although initially met with skepticism, his idea was not devoid of scientific soundness. Research has, in fact, shown that LSD can be a very effective treatment for migraine, as indole-ring molecules can easily interact with serotonin receptors. Word of mouth quickly helped spread this alternative treatment (commonly referred to as "busting"), until other posters found that psilocybin (a psychedelic substance found in mushrooms of the *Psilocybe* species) was equally effective in stopping cluster bouts in their tracks and helped with migraine. The busting treatment was born, and using hallucinogenic tryptamines improved the lives of countless of patients struggling with cluster headaches.

Eventually, from the original board, a group of advisors and researchers emerged to champion the cause, and they created a new website to discuss and analyze reports of the treatments in the subsequent years. After more than 20 years from this initial discovery, the advocacy group Clusterbusters is now fiercely advocating the scientific and research efforts needed to fully understand how these highly controversial substances can be used to treat most primary headaches. The organization has been featured in the media, feature films, and news stories around the world and is conducting important clinical trials of indole-ring compounds for the treatment of cluster headache.

Psychedelics such as LSD and psilocybin stimulate serotoninergic and dopaminergic receptors, disrupting some neural structures within the brain that are switched on during sleep. These deeper regions of the brain are believed to be the seat of human ego, or sense of self. Hallucinogens disintegrate the boundaries of ego as it is normally perceived, distorting concepts such as space and time, and allowing the brain to establish an enhanced functional connectivity between areas to the brain that normally do not communicate. As these signals are spread, the subject experiences a broad range of abnormal sensory inputs, including vivid audiovisual synesthesia, derealization, and lucid dreaming.

Recent studies have found some evidence that LSD and psilocybin may be effective in treating cluster attacks even in subhallucinogenic doses (microdosing), terminating cluster periods and extending remission possibly by a mechanism unrelated to their hallucinogenic properties. The hallucinogen dimethyl tryptamine (DMT) has a chemical structure that is similar to the triptan sumatriptan, indicating a possible shared mechanism in preventing or stopping migraine and TACs. Combined with a plant-based monoamine oxidase inhibitor (MAOI), DMT is known as ayahuasca, a compound that has been used in religious rituals for centuries for its psychotropic properties. However, no final explanation of how the hallucinogens can stop or prevent headaches has yet been found, and further research is still needed.

Since most of these substances are illegal in most countries, their use is still frequently criticized and met with significant skepticism. Many still shun this treatment since tryptamines, aside from being illegal, have their dangers, especially in mentally unstable subjects. Yet, although having to resort to hallucinogens may seem an extreme solution, the most painful headache disorders such as cluster headache can lead patients to the brink of utter desperation. Also, many of the approved drugs used today for the management and prophylaxis of these conditions are associated with important side effects, especially at the higher doses required for the most severe cases. Tryptamines may be very effective for preventive use and, if used carefully, are normally associated with limited side effects, rivaling oxygen therapy in safety and effectiveness. The need for proper research on optimal dosage and appropriate guidelines on use of these substances is challenged by their current legal status as well as significant prejudice against the use of psychotropic substances in general. The absence of proper medical research envisaged without restrictions to determine the safest and most effective doses of hallucinogens is only preventing patients from accessing a potentially safe and effective therapy. Dire necessity forces many patients to treat themselves in secret, no matter the risks and without proper guidance from a properly qualified headache specialist. Needless to say, self-medication is even more dangerous when one has to deal with compounds that are neither controlled for their pharmaceutical purity, quantity of active substances in plant-based products, nor state of preservation. The presence of legal and social barriers against adequate research has the effect of increasing the risk of side effects and adverse reactions and decreasing patients' chances for finding the optimal dosage to achieve relief effectively.

The use of marijuana (*Cannabis spp.*) for migraine treatment is slightly less controversial because its medical use is now allowed in several states. Yet the psychotropic effects of the compound found in this plant cannot go unnoticed, so its use and any research about its potential effectiveness are likely surrounded by a certain degree of stigma and skepticism. The theory behind the action of marijuana in migraine is that the cannabinoids contained in the plant may reduce pain, nausea, and other symptoms. In humans and animals, in fact, an endocannabinoid system is in place to regulate many brain functions such as hunger, emotions, cognition, movement, and pain. This system is able to influence other relevant systems that are involved in the pathogenic mechanism of migraine, such as the serotonin, GABA, glutamate, and acetylcholine ones. Marijuana's cannabinoids should, in theory, bind to the endocannabinoid receptors modulating pain, nausea, and the other symptoms of migraine.

Despite the scientific soundness of this hypothesis, the endocannabinoid system is extremely complex and inherently adaptable, so the final modulating effects are still unclear. Other compounds such as the terpenes may also influence the chemical activity of cannabinoids (known as the entourage effect), making the pharmacology of cannabis quite complicated. While some reasons that could support the use of this plant for migraineurs exist, evidence is for the most part anecdotal. The only large study present at this time that evaluated the effectiveness of cannabis in migraine was performed in Colorado, but its quality is poor at best. Since the use of cannabis is not devoid of risks (albeit limited, especially in short-term use), more research is definitely needed before the use of this plant could be safely recommended in migraine patients.

CONTROVERSIAL THEORIES ON THE ORIGINS OF MIGRAINE PAIN

Over the last century, a considerable amount of controversy surrounded the pathogenetic mechanisms of migraine. For much of the second half of the twentieth century, the dominating theory was the so-called vascular one suggested by Graham and Wolff in 1938. Their theory focused on dilation of intracranial and extracranial vessels as the source of migraine's pain, motor, and sensory disturbances. The vascular theory was well articulated and widely accepted as the most adequate explanation of the pathophysiology of migraine. According to the vascular hypothesis, migraine has two phases. During the first one (the prodromal phase), intracranial vasospasm causes a local cerebral ischemia that triggers CSD and the associated neurologic symptoms. The second phase is characterized by compensatory vasodilation of intracranial and extracranial vessels, which is the direct cause of migraine pain. Antimigraine drugs such as ergot derivatives and triptans corroborated this hypothesis since they exerted their action through their vasoconstrictive effects.

Albeit somewhat long-lived, at the end of the last century, the vascular hypothesis was set aside in favor of the neural theory. According to this hypothesis, migraine with aura was caused by paroxysmal depolarization of cortical neurons. Since this theory was also somewhat lacking, the involvement of the trigeminovascular system was also identified as a requirement in the pathogenesis of migraine. Excess neuronal activation from serotonergic neurons would cause the abnormal hyperexcitation of the brain shown during a migraine attack, and the consequent activation of the trigeminovascular system would lead to vasodilation and pain.

Famous headache experts such as Gowers and Goadsby accepted this concept as a more viable explanation of migraine, and the vascular changes occurring during a crisis were scaled back to a simple epiphenomenon. Dilation of the cranial vessels was certainly present during a headache attack, but their involvement was now neither sufficient nor necessary to induce migraine. The vascular theory was challenged because vascular changes were not necessarily found to be related to the phase of the attack. Blood flow could, in fact, be normal or even reduced during the pain phase.

The introduction of the more recent CGRP receptor antagonists apparently substantiated this claim even further. Some of them, such as olcegepant and telcagepant, have proved effective without vascular effects; they do not cause vasoconstriction as the triptans do. However, later studies found that although they do not directly cause vessels to constrict, they antagonize the powerful vasodilating effect of CGRP, thus actively inhibiting vasodilation. While they actively reduce migraine pain by preventing the activity of this neurotransmitter, CGRP receptor antagonists may actually provide confirmation of the opposite hypothesis: that arterial dilatation is indeed important in migraine.

Other studies found relevant links between migraine and cardiovascular diseases such as ischemic and hemorrhagic stroke, hypertension, preeclampsia, and myocardial infarction. This correlation of migraine and cardiovascular disease may show that vascular changes may be a causative component in migraine rather than just an epiphenomenon. Although the involvement of central neural activity and the trigeminovascular system are now accepted as fundamental in the pathogenetic mechanism of migraine, the importance of vascular contributions is a highly controversial object of debate even today.

CONCLUSION

As with many other less-understood diseases, headache diagnosis and management are surrounded by debate and diverging opinions. This chapter focused on the more controversial aspects of living with headache, its treatment, and its pathogenetic origins.

In the next chapter we will have a look at what the future (and to some extent, the present) holds for headache patients in terms of improved therapies and diagnostic aids.

10

Current Research and Future Directions

Do not undervalue the headache. While it is at its sharpest it seems a bad investment. But when relief begins, the unexpired remainder is worth $4 a minute.

—Mark Twain

As our understanding of the disease improves, headache treatment, prevention, and diagnosis keep evolving at a steady pace. This chapter will highlight the areas of current research, the latest, most important medical discoveries, and how our approach to this condition may change in the next few years.

INVASIVE NEUROMODULATION TECHNIQUES

Neuromodulation is an emerging therapeutic approach that involves the direct stimulation of a nerve or brain nucleus to normalize its physiologic activity. A stimulus that can be electrical, magnetic, or chemical in nature is applied to a target neurological site in the body, influencing the body's natural response and inducing nerve cell activity. The release of neurotransmitters and other electrophysiological effects on neural membranes is supposed to modulate aberrant or abnormal nerve tissue function, normalizing its activity from the state of perturbation. When pharmaceutical therapy has failed (such as in medication-refractory migraine, cluster headache, and trigeminal neuralgia) and surgery is not feasible or is unwanted, both invasive and noninvasive neuromodulation techniques can be tried to treat severe, chronic, or otherwise intractable primary headaches.

Invasive neuromodulation techniques are currently being researched in clinical trials and include occipital nerve stimulation (ONS), sphenopalatine ganglion (SPG) stimulation, high cervical spinal cord stimulation (SCS), and deep-brain stimulation (DBS). Wire electrodes are placed around cervical dorsal nerves from the back of the neck region in ONS or through the back of the mouth—under the cheek of the upper jaw—in SPG stimulation, and connected to a trial stimulator. In DBS, a medical device called a neurostimulator is implanted inside the brain to send electrical impulses to the hypothalamus. In this case, the rationale is that since it has been observed that the posterior hypothalamus is activated during a cluster headache attack, inhibitory high-frequency stimulation could stop the pain. In all cases, when the headache pain starts, an electrical stimulation sent by the neuromodulating device to the target area is supposed to turn the pain off. Placebo controls are made by randomly applying sham stimulation, subperception stimulation, or full stimulation doses in equal proportions. If the experiment is successful, the electrodes are thus connected to a permanently implantable pulse generator.

Recent studies have shown that ONS is able to normalize the metabolism of several pain-processing brain regions that showed hypermetabolic activity before treatment. However, ONS does not normalize hypermetabolism in the hypothalamic regions known to be involved in the generation of cluster attacks. Possibly because of this lack of effect on the hypothalamus, cluster attacks tend to recur shortly after cessation of peripheral stimulation. For migraine prevention, instead, the effectiveness of ONS is at best modest or not significant. Adverse reactions including pain, infections, and lead migrations are very common as well and, coupled with the high cost, make the widespread use of this technique largely infeasible.

For SPG stimulation, patients experience sensory disturbances in the vast majority of cases, as well as many other common side effects such as facial, nose, or mouth pain; swelling; and dry eyes. SPG stimulation has been tried for migraine treatments, with somewhat poor or inconclusive results. In any case, to date only a relatively small number of patients treated with ONS and SPG have been reported, and more data are required. High cervical SCS has shown some promise but has been tested so far in a single retrospective study of just 17 patients. A possible advantage of the high-stimulation frequency of this particular device is that it may avoid the paresthesias caused by other implantable neurostimulators, but it was never tested in randomized placebo-controlled trials.

DBS has been tested exclusively in the most severe medication-refractory chronic cluster headache patients only. In particular, it has been used in patients suffering from daily or almost daily attacks for least one or two years. Deep hypothalamic stimulation was already used in some chronic patients who obtained persistent pain reduction or abolition after a four-year follow-up. Although DBS eventually became ineffective for some of them, despite many changes in the stimulation settings, their headache improved from the intractable chronic form to a typical episodic form characterized by long periods of complete remission. Interestingly enough, during one clinical trial, active DBS stimulation provided no benefits over sham stimulation during the first month of therapy. However, by the end of the one-year open-label phase, nearly half of the patients had achieved at least a 50% reduction in cluster attack frequency, showing how this type of therapy might require some time before becoming effective. Just like the other types of neuromodulation, DBS has been tested so far on a relatively small number of patients, and more studies are, therefore, required before this rather drastic measure could be recommended.

NONINVASIVE NEUROMODULATION TECHNIQUES

To avoid the risks associated with surgery and invasive implantation of neurostimulators, new, noninvasive techniques to modulate pain are currently being researched and tested. Effective neuromodulation can be achieved even by stimulating the nervous system centrally or at the periphery by applying an electrical current or a fluctuating magnetic field through the skin. Interestingly enough, these approaches can have both immediate and long-term effects, making them suitable for both abortive treatment of acute attacks as well as prophylactic therapy.

Although noninvasive neuromodulation techniques show much promise, the randomized placebo-controlled trials completed to date are still very few, and questions have been raised about the degree of blinding of some of them. Caution must therefore be exercised before recommending them, and prudence would dictate reservation until more evidence is published.

Noninvasive Vagus-Nerve Stimulation (nVNS)

Vagus-nerve stimulation (VNS) was originally devised as an invasive treatment of refractory epilepsy and depression. Anecdotal observation of improvement in migraine patients treated with the early implantable devices led to the exploration of less invasive systems. Noninvasive vagus-nerve stimulation (nVNS) is achieved through a small, handheld electrical stimulator that is placed on the skin and delivers a transcutaneous current to the cervical branch of the vagus nerve. The device (known as gammaCore®) can be easily operated by the patients several times per day to abort migraine and cluster headache attacks, and it produces a short-lasting, little tingling sensation. Beyond the advantage of not having to undergo surgery, this nVNS system allows patients to put it on themselves, vastly improving treatment adherence to achieve effective migraine prevention without the use of drugs. The exact mechanism by which nVNS could help in migraine treatment is, however, unknown. A possible explanation is that it could exert a downstream modulatory effect on the nucleus tractus solitarius, which has projections to some of the central regions involved in the genesis of headache, such as the thalamus, hypothalamus, reticular activating system, amygdala/hippocampus, cerebral cortex, and trigeminal nucleus caudalis.

Although many smaller studies showed promising results in terms of reduction in the frequency of attacks and high tolerability of the device, the only randomized controlled study to test the efficacy of nVNS in migraine prevention to date has failed to show a significant difference between active and sham treatment. Initial reporting from large studies suggested, instead, that VNS could have a greater potential in the prophylactic and acute treatment of chronic cluster. Common adverse events include stiff neck, frequent urination, shoulder pain or spasm, lip or facial drooping, neck twitching, and raspy voice. Another VNS device known as the Nemos® device has been developed to stimulate the aurical branch of the vagus nerve by having users wear the electrode in the ear. However, current data are not yet sufficient to support its regular use in clinical practice.

Transcutaneous Cranial Nerve Stimulation

Transcutaneous supraorbital nerve stimulation (STS) and transcutaneous occipital nerve stimulation (tONS) are two forms of transcutaneous electrical stimulation of the cranial nerves. The supraorbital branch of the trigeminal nerve is responsible for providing sensation to the forehead and upper eyelid. It has hypothesized that transcutaneous stimulation of these nerves could modulate pain by inhibiting nociceptive transmission in small pain-transmitting fibers, thus providing benefit during migraine attacks. STS has been studied for the prevention of episodic migraine in a first multicenter, randomized, sham-controlled, double-blind clinical trial of 67 patients and later in a large, open-label study of 2,313 headache sufferers who could rent the stimulator via the internet for 40 days.

The most frequently reported side effect was mild and fully reversible paresthesia in the area of stimulation, which could be intolerable in some and lead to interruption. It has also caused a certain degree of unblinding during the randomized controlled trial. Arousal and sleep changes were the second most common adverse events. So far, the results of STS have been positive, with a 30% reduction in migraine days and a 26% therapeutic gain over the sham treatment. The same device used for STS can be used for tONS and, so far, has shown promising results compared with sham stimulation and 100 milligrams topiramate daily in 110 subjects. Research on combined occipital and supraorbital transcutaneous nerve stimulation with an OSTNS neurostimulator is currently ongoing.

Transcranial Magnetic Stimulation (TMS)

Single-pulse transcranial magnetic stimulation (TMS) is a magnetic device that has been used in the field of neuroscience for decades, albeit for different uses. Since 2014, it was approved by the U.S. Food and Drug Administration as a safe, noninvasive alternative for migraine treatment and prevention. The TMS device is a magnet placed at the back of the head for less than a minute by the patient to generate a single magnetic pulse. It acts by creating a fluctuating magnetic field that induces a mild electric current at the back of the brain. This electric current does not cause any discomfort and is believed to modify the excitability of cortical neurons inhibiting cortical spreading depression and to prevent thalamocortical circuits from firing pain signals. This activity supposedly "turns off" migraine attacks and is also effective in migraine prophylaxis. The patient turns on the TMS device by pressing a button, and the pulses generated can be self-administered to stop an attack or can be repeated as prescribed by a neurologist to reduce the frequency of attacks.

Two large studies in both the United Kingdom and the United States have shown promising results in the acute treatment of migraine, although the results are still inconclusive as to the efficacy of TMS for the preventive treatment of this condition. A +17% therapeutic gain over sham treatment has been estimated, and minimal adverse events (usually headache, migraine, and sinusitis) have been reported in just 5% of patients (against 2% in sham stimulation subjects). The absence of serious side effects, together with additional pharmacoeconomic studies, suggests that TMS is a safe and cost-effective alternative for migraine patients, although larger, postmarketing trials to evaluate it in the long term are still ongoing.

Other Noninvasive Neuromodulation Techniques

Additional noninvasive neuromodulation techniques have been explored, although all these methods have only been tested in a very small group of patients.

In transcranial direct current stimulation experiments, an anodal (excitatory) or cathodal (inhibitory) electric current is applied to the scalp to modulate cortical excitability. The theory is that this current could prevent or stop migraine attacks by modifying the potential of underlying cortical neurons. Cathodal inhibitory currents have, so far, failed to show any appreciable effect in migraine treatment or prevention. Anodal activating currents, instead, proved to be effective in reducing attack frequency and pain intensity, but results were only seen at 4 and 8 weeks after treatment and not at 12 weeks, suggesting a possible short-term effect.

In percutaneous mastoid electrical stimulation (PMES) an electric current is administered behind the ear through the skin to stimulate the fastigial nucleus of the cerebellum. The neuroprotective effect of PMES has already been subject to experiment against cerebral ischemia, and a recent randomized, double-blind, sham-controlled trial explored its application in migraine prevention. Although the higher response rate (50%) in the treatment group is very encouraging, the actual blinding degree in this study can hardly be assessed, and more evidence is certainly needed.

In nonpainful brachial electric stimulation, the electrical current is applied on the arm rather than on the head, neck, or back. A very discrete armband that delivers the electrical current is worn under clothing by patients, who can control it through an app installed on their smartphones. A small prospective, randomized, double-blind, sham-controlled, crossover trial explored the effectiveness of this treatment for acute treatment of migraine, with mixed results. The therapeutic gain over sham stimulation was quite modest, and 39% of patients rated active stimulation as either painful or unpleasant.

Calcitonin Gene–Related Peptide (CGRP) Receptor Antagonists and Monoclonal Antibodies

Calcitonin gene–related peptide (CGRP) is a neuropeptide produced in both peripheral and central neurons with potent vasodilator properties at the cerebral artery level. CGRP is found in both unmyelinated and thinly myelinated fibers throughout the trigeminal nerve system. It is also found in the trigeminocervical complex and in other regions of the central nervous system. Recent studies have identified CGRP as a potential candidate in migraine therapy due to the role of this neuropeptide in modulating central and peripheral pain circuits. During migraine attacks, jugular levels of CGRP have found to be increased, and intravenous administration of this peptide induces a headache in most migraine patients. CGRP may have a regulatory function in the transmission of central nociception, and an increase in levels of this molecule in migraineurs is associated with reduced descending inhibitory mechanisms that could lead to headache sensitivity. The CGRP pathway is, therefore, becoming an emerging target for the development of new drugs that act as antagonists of its receptor (CGRPR).

The first class of drugs developed as CGRPR antagonists are the gepants, a group of nonpeptide small molecules effective for use in acute migraine. These molecules can abort migraine attacks without having vasoconstrictor effects, making them useful in patients for whom triptans are contraindicated, such as those who have angina, hypertension, peripheral vascular disease, or other vascular diseases. Most studies have reported positive outcomes in terms of pain freedom and an acceptable side effects profile. However, two studies, including one on telcagepant, were stopped due to liver toxicity, and three others because of lack of interest from the pharmaceutical companies. Both ubrogepant and rimegepant received approval from the FDA for the acute treatment of migraine, in December 2019 and February 2020, respectively.

Another group of effective and well-tolerated drugs that have been recently approved for preventive use in migraine and cluster headache is represented by monoclonal antibodies (mAbs) targeting either the CGRP peptide itself (galcanezumab, fremanezumab, and eptinezumab) or its canonical receptor (erenumab). Anti-CGRP mAbs remove excess CGRP molecules, while anti-CGRP receptor mAbs block signaling at the receptor. By weakening or preventing the activation of the CGRP signaling pathway, the frequency of headaches is reduced over time. These molecules have been approved for medical use in the United States and in some countries in the European Union between 2018 and 2020. All the mABs demonstrated a good safety, tolerability, and efficacy profile in migraine patients, and galcanezumab was the first monoclonal antibody approved in the United States for the treatment of episodic cluster headache in adults. Erenumab, galcanezumab, and fremanezumab are all administered by subcutaneous injection once per month, while eptinezumab is administered by intravenous infusion once every three months. Their side effects mostly consist of pain and redness at the site of the injection and may include allergic reactions. The real limit to the use of these molecules is their elevated cost. Their use is therefore justified only when it's counterbalanced by a high patient benefit, such as in very severe or therapy-refractory patients.

Other targets for migraine therapy have identified other neurotransmitters and their receptors involved in neuroinflammatory mechanisms, such as substance P, neurokinin 1, orexin, and NO. Clinical trials, however, have consistently failed to demonstrate any effectiveness in treatment or prophylaxis of headaches, diminishing any initial enthusiasm. The only other treatment that so far has demonstrated any activity in several nonclinical studies in migraine prophylaxis is the intranasal administration of oxyto-cin, a natural hormone that could block the release of the CGRP. Larger, double-blind, placebo-controlled clinical trials are, however, still necessary to properly assess its effectiveness and safety.

Novel Drug Delivery Systems

Although triptans still remain the mainstay therapy for acute treatment of migraine and cluster headache, new routes of drug administrations have improved the quality of treatment. Like all oral medications, triptan tab-lets are also subject to gastrointestinal and hepatic first-pass metabolism, which reduces their bioavailability to about 15% in humans. Because of that, approximately one-third of patients in clinical trials fail to obtain headache relief with oral sumatriptan medications. The new delivery sys-tems can skip the gastrointestinal system, allowing for lower doses to be used and circumventing further issues with absorption, such as those caused by gastroparesis, nausea, and vomit.

Sumatriptan, the oldest available drug in this category, has been recently proposed in new delivery formulations that maximize its efficacy and effectiveness, reduce the time before pain relief is achieved, and minimize adverse reactions and side effects. While subcutaneous injections are a valid alternative to oral administration, they are associated with a substan-tial rate of injection-site reactions and triptan-associated side effects. The nose has been identified as an attractive delivery route, since the richly vascularized mucosal surface is perfectly suited for rapid absorption of medications into the systemic circulation. While interesting, the applica-tion of a conventional triptan nasal spray has been limited since the intense bitter taste of the liquid often discourages use in many patients. Also, a large percentage of the dose administered is actually swallowed, becom-ing, in effect, an orally administered medication with all the disadvantages noted previously.

Much more technologically advanced than the liquid spray, a newer, breath-powered sumatriptan dry nasal powder administered through an intranasal device has been recently approved for the general market. While this advanced system is actually not a true nasal spray, it is often referred to as such, generating some confusion. This new device is placed inside the nostril, but the drug is actually activated by exhaling when a fine powder reaches the upper nasal cavity. As the soft palate is closed, the nasal cavity is expanded, and the nasal device delivers the powdered triptan that adheres to the moist nasal mucosa. The nasal route has the advantage of a speedy onset, since pain relief usually occurs very rapidly, requiring as lit-tle as 15 minutes for some patients. For this reason, the breath-powered system has been proposed as a valid alternative to subcutaneous injectable sumatriptan for the control of acute cluster headache attacks.

Another very modern device is an iontophoretic transdermal patch delivery system that is applied to the skin to deliver sumatriptan. A minuscule electrical current allows the drug to cross the skin barrier and get absorbed into the bloodstream, circumventing the gastrointestinal system and allowing for a lower dose to be released. The device is applied on the upper arm or the thigh, and it's activated with a button. A small battery is required to provide the electrical current. The main advantage of this device is that it maintains a constant delivery of small doses of sumatriptan over a period of four hours, minimizing side effects and maximizing its efficacy over time. Although pain relief may require some time to be fully reached, nausea is usually eliminated within one to two hours. This drug delivery system is a good alternative for patients suffering from severe nausea or vomiting who cannot ingest tablets. It is also helpful for those who cannot tolerate triptan-related adverse events, or those with a suboptimal response to oral medications.

CONCLUSION

Luckily enough, the future seems to hold much promise for headache patients in terms of new treatments, drugs, and modern therapeutic approaches. In this chapter we discussed the newest medications available or currently being tested for treating and preventing major headaches, as well as the latest therapeutic solutions, such as neuromodulation techniques and novel drug delivery systems.

In the next section of the book, we use some sample stories to illustrate some aspects of the diseases that we have already discussed in the preceding chapters. These fictional stories will let the reader explore the challenges and hardships of living with a headache, obtaining an initial diagnosis, dealing with the possible complications, observing possible effects on family and friends, and so on.

Case Illustrations

CLUSTER HEADACHE: THE INFAMOUS "SUICIDE HEADACHE"

Darren is a 34-year-old man. During his adolescence, he suffered from tremendous headaches that woke him up at night, lasted for nearly an hour, and left him fatigued for several hours after they were over. For months, he tried all kinds of OTC medications to make them stop: from aspirin to ibuprofen and even caffeine tablets, but the headaches kept waking him up, screaming in pain, nearly every night. After many medical tests, checks and visits to different specialists (general practitioner, oculist, neurologist, just to name a few), an otolaryngologist diagnosed him with a sinusitis caused by cold. Shortly after that visit, the headache disappeared completely, leaving Darren free for many years until he forgot about it entirely.

But sadly for Darren, the headache came back again when he was 21, this time becoming much more frequent and painful. The pain seemed to drill down inside one side of the poor guy's skull, irradiating toward the mandible and behind the ear and reaching unbearable levels. Attacks woke him up at night, just like last time, but they also came back during the day, usually at around the same hour, and lasted for 30–90 minutes. Darren tried the medications prescribed to him for sinusitis to no avail; he was left racked by a brutal pain that seemingly never left him able to work or even get out of his house. Shortly before scheduling a surgical intervention of rhinoplasty, though, a friend of Darren's referred him to a neurologist who specialized in headaches, who quickly recognized the patterns of a very typical cluster headache. After a short course of steroids, the pain subsided, and the bout disappeared in a few weeks.

Eventually, Darren learned much about his condition, its patterns, and the correct therapies. As soon as the pain came back during the winter months, he immediately started his treatment with verapamil, slowly increasing the dosage to avoid a risk of adverse cardiovascular reactions. For the next 10 years, things seemed under control. Between verapamil, steroids, and occasional shots of intramuscular sumatriptan, Darren was able to keep the cluster controlled and live a normal life. However, once he hit 30, the situation started to rapidly decline. He could not tolerate verapamil at the dosage that he needed; it caused him to suffer from low blood pressure and constant fatigue, and he often fainted. His cardiologist advised him not to increase the dose further, though Darren's pain was unbearable. The medication reduced his attacks from four per day to just two, one of which was during the night. But since the dose was not high enough, the nightly attack could last up to two and a half hours, leaving him devastated. Nor was the sumatriptan injection an option anymore, as he could not use it every day due to its high cost and consistent side effects.

Darren cannot sleep, work, or function well anymore. He lives in constant fear of the next attack and now has trouble even coping with the fear. While looking for solutions on the internet, he found Clusterbusters. org, an important resource for "clusterheads," where he now meets many fellow patients. Here he finds out about the "Vitamin M" treatment—a therapy consisting of the administration of psilocybin mushrooms to "break" the cluster. He's got no alternatives and wants to try it, but he doesn't know where to find those mushrooms, since they're illegal in the United States. He finally finds a friend of a friend who sells them, but when he does buy them, he can't help but feel like a junkie. He tries them a couple of times with great results, nearly achieving his goal to break the cluster. However, the fourth time he tries them, the mushrooms have spoiled, and he ends up vomiting a lot, feeling bad for days, and ending up in the emergency room. As soon as they find out he's been hospitalized for toxic substances poisoning, his wife and his relatives question his choice, wondering why he's resorting to illegal drugs to treat his headache. Word of mouth runs quickly, and eventually his boss finds out and decides to fire him, thinking he's a good-for-nothing dealing with a drug addiction. Darren's life seems ruined, and he's left stranded and alone, struggling with pain, and without any chance to get the only treatment that was effective for him. Now he fully understands why this headache is called "suicide headache." The community at Clusterbusters.org, however, proves to be immensely helpful. Its members teach him about other alternatives for his condition and help him enroll for a clinical trial to experiment with monoclonal antibodies.

Analysis

Cluster headache is one of the most painful conditions known in medicine (see chapters 1 and 4). This case study has shown that psychedelics may be the only therapeutic alternative for patients forced to endure this inhumane pain and that this choice is often met with skepticism or outright rejection by society (chapter 9).

One of the greatest challenges to receiving a proper diagnosis of cluster headache, especially in its early stages, is its circannual periodicity (chapter 5). When Darren had his first cluster bout during his adolescence, he did not, in fact, receive a correct diagnosis but was diagnosed with sinusitis, as is often the case for cluster headache patients (chapter 7). However, the cluster eventually subsided on its own, leaving him with the false reassurance that the first treatment course, for sinusitis, was the right one. It would take more years of pain and wrong treatment for the patient to eventually realize that that diagnosis was wrong in the first place.

When Darren finally finds a treatment, however, things improve just for a short period. Cluster headache is an insidious disease that often becomes refractory to treatment over time (chapter 5), leaving him very few options. Darren tries a controversial solution (chapter 9), but while the treatment can be effective, without proper medical support or standardized pharmacological substances available, his situation doesn't improve. Luckily for him, the research never stops, so he can enroll in a clinical trial and test some of the latest drugs available (chapter 10).

SURVIVING MIGRAINE: A DIFFICULT LIFE

Herbert is a 28-year-old cook from Boston who suffers from a very persistent and ruinous headache. Sometimes he wakes up in the morning feeling uneasy, his head heavy and his thoughts clouded. Within a few hours the head pain becomes stronger, throbbing, and he starts to feel nauseous. Every sound, every smell of the restaurant's kitchen where he works become unbearable—all stimuli only make him feel worse. He would just like to isolate himself in a dark, silent room, but he's often required to keep working. He ends up vomiting from time to time to find some respite.

Herbert can't remember the first time he suffered from these headaches. He was probably young, probably in his early teens, but it was during adolescence that they became stronger and more frequent. Herbert's mother suffered from a similar fate, and he remembers her spending entire days writhing in pain in her bedroom. Eventually he was diagnosed with migraine, and his therapy consisted of a triptan to take whenever he felt too bad.

Herbert has recently accepted a new job in a very crowded restaurant in San Francisco. The wages are nearly twice as high as at his previous job, but he's had to move to the other side of the country, which was a challenge his wife and kids eagerly accepted with the prospect of a better life. However, changing the time zone wreaked havoc on his habits, making his migraine more frequent and painful than ever. He tries to "man up," but the triptans sometimes do not even kick in anymore, and he needs to work at a frantic pace to keep up with the needs of the new kitchen he now manages. To add insult to injury, when the weekend finally comes, the migraines often strike with a vengeance, forcing him to lie down on the bed or couch for two days in a row.

Amanda, Herbert's wife, is tired of all this. She left her previous job in Boston to follow him, and during the week she now takes care of the home and their two kids, Bertha and Jeffrey. Needless to say, she eagerly waits all week to spend some time with her husband, but most of the time, she has to take care of him, as he's too plagued by the migraines to even move. She and Herbert often fight because of this, causing him to feel tremendous pressure. Herbert has tried to explain his situation to his boss, hoping to find a solution that allows him to work in somewhat less stressful conditions, albeit at reduced pay. Herbert's boss, however, is inflexible. The boss says he'll have to find another cook if Herbert's not up for the task, as the needs of the restaurants must come first.

Things go completely south when Amanda's parents plan to come to visit for her birthday. She wants to throw a huge party with her family to celebrate his father's recent victory against cancer—the poor man was successfully diagnosed cancer free after a long chemotherapy treatment cycle. She planned the event well ahead, asking Herbert to help her, but when the time comes, Herbert is struck by a humongous migraine that does not stop even after he takes a double dose of rizatriptan. A huge fight ensues in front of the whole family; ultimately, the woman leaves the house for good and goes back to Boston. As Herbert struggles to keep his job no matter what, he now has to deal with all the hardships of an impending divorce. He wonders how it can be his fault that he's been cursed with this disease.

Analysis

If not properly treated, even the simplest migraine may have a tremendous impact on the quality of life of a patient affected by it (chapter 6) and can negatively impact the patient's family as well. This case focused on the socioeconomic burden of this condition on the patient and his family and on how frequently migraine can damage a patient's life well beyond the pain and physical symptoms (chapters 6 and 7).

Migraine is a complex neurological condition that goes well beyond the definition of a simple "headache" (chapter 1). Herbert's mother suffered from migraine as well; no surprise there, as this condition frequently runs in families due to its possible genetic origin (chapters 1 and 3). Herbert's migraine seems to have worsened with his move. The worsening of this condition is often associated with drastic lifestyle changes and stress, among other triggers (chapter 3). Stress seems to be a major issue in this case, and as it further aggravates the disease, it brings more stress, generating a vicious cycle. In fact, he even suffers from the dreaded "weekend headache" or "letdown migraine" (chapter 8). Herbert's migraine is not adequately managed, though; he would probably benefit from a prophylactic therapy since his attacks are so frequent and have started to not respond to triptans (chapter 8).

Eventually, migraine degrades Herbert's quality of life to a point of no return, as his wife and family cannot cope with the burden of living with a migraine patient anymore (chapter 7).

TENSION HEADACHE AND MEDICATION OVERUSE: WHEN LESS IS ACTUALLY MORE

Clare is a 45-year-old woman from New York. She is a very busy data analyst who often spends her time working all day long for a big marketing agency. For most of her life, Clare has never suffered from significant headache but just the occasional one she would treat with an OTC medication. Lately, though, her headaches have become more than just a nuisance. They have become extremely frequent and often last long enough and are heavy enough to force her to stop working altogether—something that has never happened to her before. Her pain is like a tight band around her head, irradiating to the neck, and is often accompanied by nausea and numbness in her fingers. Sometimes, when the headache is really strong, she almost can't feel her hands anymore.

Clare has asked her doctor for a remedy, but the clinician quickly dismissed her, telling her that it was just a minor ailment—nothing to be worried about. "Everyone suffers from headache from time to time. Don't be a whiner, and endure them," he told Clare, and he recommended that she take aspirin and drink plenty of water to feel better. Clare has been following the advice, but as time goes on, the headaches are becoming stronger, longer, and more riddled with complications. After talking with a friend about her issue, Clare decides to see a neurologist who specializes in headaches. After a brief visit, the neurologist advises her to start taking notes on her headaches and the medication she takes, so she can have a better understanding of what causes her headaches and how frequent they are.

After a few weeks of writing her headache diary, Clare realizes that her headaches become more frequent when her workload is particularly heavy, so she decides to take a break for a few days. Her minivacation makes her feel better, but she still suffers from many headaches. After confronting her neurologist about that, he checks her headache diary to see if he can spot something else. The neurologist actually realizes that Clare has taken an aspirin nearly every other day in the last three months, and while it was effective in the beginning, now it's only making her feeling worse. Before he attempts any other diagnosis, he decides that Clare must get rid of her NSAID medications for a while, and he gives her a course of amitriptyline to help her cope with the withdrawal symptoms.

After three weeks, Clare feels better, but the original headache still haunts her. After discussing it a bit more, the neurologist refers her to a radiologist to get an X-ray scan of her neck. The radiologist quickly finds out what the issue is: Clare has a restriction in her cervical vertebrae, so the headache may be caused by an improper seating posture and aggravated when she must work a lot. He suggests Clare do some physical exercise to strengthen her neck and back muscles, improve her posture while seating, and buy a new, more ergonomic chair. Clare follows his advice, and in a few weeks her headaches subside, finally leaving her pain free for the first time in a long time.

Analysis

This case explored the usual vicious cycle where a patient affected by recurring musculoskeletal headaches ends up taking NSAIDs too frequently until the headache itself is caused by the medications rather than by the underlying condition (chapter 1). Clare's symptoms closely resemble a tension-type headache (TTH), as can be deduced by the late emergence of the condition and the extremely suggestive description of the "tight band around the head" (chapter 4). However, when it comes to TTH, it's easy for both patients and health-care providers to underestimate the severity of the condition (chapter 1).

When the neurologist visits Clare, he tries to identify the root causes of her headache by asking her to write a headache diary. Headache diaries are an extremely useful diagnostic tool that also help patients improve their awareness and understanding of their condition (chapter 8). In this situation, Clare must deal with a medication-overuse headache (MOH) first and foremost, so her neurologist prescribes her a neuroleptic to help her deal with the withdrawal stage (chapter 5). Once the MOH issue is finally resolved, additional tests will identify the cause of Clare's TTH, which seems to be linked with an underlying neck issue (chapter 3). To some extent, Clare's TTH can be considered a secondary headache (chapter 1). In any case, appropriate lifestyle interventions seem enough to finally provide her relief from her pain, leading to a positive outcome (chapter 6).

PEDIATRIC HEADACHES: ALL'S WELL THAT ENDS WELL

Martin has suffered from headaches since his early childhood. He can't really remember when he had his first attack. He only remembers his mother screaming at him because he didn't want to go to school again. "I'm tired of your tantrums! You're just a whiny brat and a wimp! You're scared to go to school; I don't want to hear your excuses anymore!" Yet Martin's pain wasn't a lie—the poor boy really was plagued by constant headaches and not just when he had to go to school. It wasn't so rare for him to end up throwing up his lunch after he spent all his afternoon doing his homework. At some point, his parents decided to bring him to the doctor, who referred him to an oculist, who claimed it was just some eyestrain, even though he had no sight problems whatsoever. His life wasn't simple at school either, as Martin was often bullied by his peers, who saw him as a "weakling" who suffered from some psychological weakness.

Martin had to spend many more years plagued by his problem before his family decided to take the matter more seriously. His life took a turn when he was 13, though, when he experienced something that scared him and his relatives. All of a sudden, during dinner, he started seeing a blinding light. After that, his vision blurred almost entirely, except for a small "hole" in the middle of his eyes. He couldn't see anything beyond that for several hours, and his parents brought him to the emergency room thinking he was having a stroke. Instead, it was just a migraine aura, as the knowledgeable neurologist quickly found out. Martin was prescribed some abortive medications, but while these helped him feel better physically, his social situation didn't improve.

On the contrary, Martin had to deal with the hardships of being a teenager with migraine now. Every time he tried to stay up late, he had a tremendous headache that lasted for the whole next day, but his friends told him it was just a "hangover." He was banned from drinking alcohol, as it would worsen his condition, but that led to his friends teasing him for being a "wimp." It didn't take long before everyone at school, not just his friends, started mocking Martin, the timid kid who didn't want to drink alcohol and stay up late at night.

Eventually school was over, but life wasn't easy for Martin even after that. To pay for his university expenses, he took a job at a famous fast-food chain. Sometimes he just felt too bad to go to work, and after a few absences, his boss didn't want to hear any more excuses and laid him off.

Even when Martin showed his boss a medical certificate that proved he suffered from migraine, his former boss scoffed at him and called him a "girlie." He told Martin that "migraine is a disease for women" and that he had to man up and endure the attacks.

However, after Martin turned 19, and after many struggles, his life seemed to gradually improve. The migraines have gradually subsided on their own, without any particular intervention on Martin's part, leaving him plenty of time and space to enjoy his hobbies and passions. Eventually, he became completely headache free. When he becomes a successful adult, Martin will be able to set migraine aside as a (bad) memory of the past.

Analysis

It's often hard to detect and diagnose migraines and other severe headaches in children, let alone manage them adequately. This case explored the challenges of dealing with migraine from childhood, as well as the social stigma associated with this condition (chapter 7).

Martin's headache was clearly a migraine even during childhood, as suggested by many details (chapter 4). For example, his headache was more frequent in the morning (he didn't want to go to school). It became worse after he spent an afternoon studying (stress and eyestrain), to the extent that he ended up vomiting (a typical autonomic symptom of this condition). However, as it often happens with childhood headaches, it was largely underestimated by his family, who took his attacks for mere tantrums (chapter 7). However, childhood headaches are a serious issue that represent the third most frequent cause of school absenteeism (chapter 6).

Martin's story also highlights an issue that is common with many primary headaches: the very long time required (years in this case) before a patient can finally receive a proper diagnosis (chapter 1). In this case, Martin only got a diagnosis when his symptoms seemingly mimicked a more serious underlying cerebrovascular disease (chapters 4 and 5). However, it was just a misunderstanding that frequently occurred when a patient experienced a migraine aura for the first time (chapter 4).

Though he now has a diagnosis, Martin must deal with many limitations that impact his quality of life quite significantly (chapter 6). Drinking alcohol or losing sleep, while normal things for teenagers, can be powerful triggers for migraine (chapter 3). Both during his adolescence and his early adulthood, Martin must face the challenging barriers and the severe stigma associated with migraine (chapter 9). Probably the most ridiculous insult he has to endure is being called a "girl." While it is true that migraine affects more women than men (chapter 6), the stigma associated with being a male individual affected by migraine has never died, despite having its historical roots in previous centuries (chapter 2).

Luckily for Martin, though, childhood migraine is usually associated with a good prognosis, and as soon as he reached adulthood, his headache went into complete remission (chapter 6).

HEADACHES AND PSYCHOLOGICAL ISSUES: THE PROBLEM IS INSIDE MY HEAD

Amelia is a woman with a sad past. A few years ago, when she was younger, she met Adrian, a strong-handed ambulance driver with a somewhat rough personality. The two quickly fell in love and married soon thereafter, giving birth to a daughter, Samantha. However, Adrian was a violent man, and on many occasions, Amelia had to deal with his angry outbursts that frequently ended with physical violence. One day, Amelia decided that Adrian's last violent outburst was the last straw. When she threatened to leave him, Adrian overreacted, and in a quick escalation of events, he ended up taking his rage out against their daughter as well. When the police came, they found Amelia unconscious in a pool of blood, but unfortunately for the little Sammy, there was nothing to be done. Adrian killed himself shortly after taking their daughter's life, and needless to say, Amelia was left deeply traumatized.

In the subsequent years, Amelia needed the help of several psychologists to overcome her tremendous trauma, but as a sort of side effect of these terrible events, she now suffers from frequent recurring headaches. These headaches are hard to describe: the pain is diffusely distributed across the entire skull and often associated with a generalized sensation of malaise and fatigue. She's had a very hard time finding a job and starting a new life, as these headaches seemingly prevent her from doing much, often start as soon as she wakes up, and last for the entire day. After all the horrific events she had to go through, Amelia was left scarred and is now suspicious about all things medical, as they somehow remind her of Adrian. Therefore, she refuses to take any medication to treat her disease beyond sertraline, the antidepressant she absolutely needs to cope with her never-ending anxiety.

Looking on the internet for some "natural remedy," she finds out about St. John's wort, an herb that many people claim to be very effective against headaches. She proceeds to purchase some capsules of this herbal remedy online, but her results are mixed at best. After talking with some random strangers in a social media group called "Natural Medicine," she decides that the dosage of herb contained in those capsules was too low to be effective and tries to double it without talking with her doctor. A few hours after she took the third dose, she starts feeling really hot, her heart is racing, and her forehead is dripping with sweat. Agitated, she calls emergency services, who treat her for serotonin syndrome.

After a couple of days of observation, Amelia is discharged from the hospital and sent back to her psychiatrist, who advises her to start CBT and switches her to a different antidepressant, amitriptyline. Amelia takes her doctor's advice reluctantly and starts the therapy. As the counseling sessions go on, the therapist finds new ways to help her cope with her past issues and the anxiety she suffers from. The therapist also advises her to go to the gym, as physical exercise could help her improve her mood, and gives her some magnesium supplements to "calm her nerves." She gradually learns to deal with her anxiety, and her headaches improve as well, slowly becoming less and less frequent over time.

Analysis

This case focused on the psychological comorbidities of headache and the relative value of nonpharmacological approaches. Amelia must deal with the ghosts of a traumatizing past, and she now suffers from anxiety and post-traumatic stress disorder (PTSD). Following the *ICHD*-3 guidelines (chapter 2), her headache could be classified as "Headache attributed to psychiatric disorder." Her headaches can arguably be caused by her psychological issues, although it's hard to be sure whether they are truly secondary headaches or not (chapter 1). It is possible that she's just suffering from a TTH that is worsened by her psychiatric comorbidity, as she's often very stressed by her mental anguish (chapter 8). In any case, headaches are frequently comorbid with several psychiatric conditions such as depression, anxiety, and mood disorders, and the cause-effect association between these two disease categories often goes both ways (chapter 6).

Not trusting pharmacological therapy to treat her headaches, Amelia chooses to try a natural remedy, St. John's wort, which is known to be effective. However, doing so without medical supervision can be very dangerous. *Hypericum perforatum*, in fact, is a potent monoamine oxidase inhibitor (MAO-I). When combined with a selective serotonin reuptake inhibitor medication such as the antidepressant she's taking (sertraline), it may lead to a serious reaction known as serotonin syndrome (chapter 5).

Thinking the true reason behind Amelia's headaches could be her anxiety and/or PTSD, her psychiatrist advises her to consult a therapist. Cognitive behavioral therapy and physical exercise could provide relief from headaches in some instances, especially when headaches are strictly associated with stress and underlying psychological issues (chapter 5). In any case, it's hard to determine what really helped Amelia in this situation. In fact, she switched her therapy and is now under treatment with amitriptyline, an antidepressant often used for preventive treatment of headaches (chapter 5). On top of that, her therapist also advised her to take a magnesium supplement, a substance that is known to be effective in preventing headaches in some patients (chapter 8).

Glossary

Abortive therapy
A therapy that aims at stopping a headache or limiting its symptoms (such as providing pain relief) once it's manifest, regardless of its ability to reduce the frequency of headache attacks.

Aura
An epiphenomenon of migraine consisting of a series of sensory disturbances that occur during the prodromal phase of the headache, shortly before an attack.

Autonomic nervous system
A component of the peripheral nervous system that regulates a broad range of involuntary body functions such as digestion, heart rate, blood pressure, breathing, and sexual arousal.

Autonomic symptom
Symptom associated with a dysfunction of the autonomic nervous system, such as nausea, vomit, runny nose, photophobia, conjunctival injection, and tachycardia, among others. It is often present in trigeminal autonomic cephalalgias and migraine.

Clusterhead
A nonderogatory slang/jargon term used to define a patient affected by cluster headache.

Cluster headache
A primary headache of the trigeminal autonomic cephalalgia (TAC) group characterized by cyclically recurrent attacks of excruciating pain.

Conjunctival injection
The enlargement of blood vessels within the eye in the conjunctiva region. It is also known as "red eye" It is an important clue used during the differential diagnosis process.

Cortical spreading depression (CSD)
A slowly propagating wave of sustained neuronal hyperactivity moving across the brain, followed by a wave of electrophysiological inhibition. It is thought to be the underlying mechanism of migraine aura.

Differential diagnosis
A process used to distinguish between the different headache disorders that may share similar clinical features.

Headache diary
A daily diary kept by headache patients to help them keep track of their attacks, symptoms, treatments, and triggers, among other pertinent data.

Hemicrania continua
A very rare and particularly disabling form of migraine characterized by continuous pain that could last for several months with no pauses between day and night.

Hypothalamus
A small region of the brain, located at its base, that is responsible for the regulation of critical metabolic and hormonal processes, circadian rhythms, and various activities of the autonomic nervous system. It is thought to play a central role in the pathogenetic mechanism of several primary headaches with a distinct cyclical recurrence, such as cluster headache.

The International Classification of Headache Disorders (ICHD)
A detailed hierarchical system that classifies and defines all known headache disorders published by the International Headache Society. It is currently available in its third iteration, the *ICHD-3*, and it is regarded as the official classification of headaches by the World Health Organization.

Medication-overuse headache (MOH)
A highly prevalent secondary headache caused by the abuse of medications used for treating headaches. Also known as "rebound headache."

Microdosing
The practice of using subthreshold doses of psychedelic drugs such as psilocybin or LSD in an attempt to abort cluster headache bouts.

Migraine
A highly prevalent, highly disabling primary headache characterized by numerous secondary symptoms, such as nausea, vomit, or hypersensitivity to sounds, odors, and lights.

Migraineur
A term used to define a patient affected by migraine.

Migrainous infarction
A rare and potentially fatal complication of migraine that occurs when migraine aura symptoms gradually worsen until they evolve into an ischemic stroke. Also known as migrainous stroke.

Neurostimulation
A medical process through which the nervous system's activity is modulated by the application of electrical or magnetic currents. It could be achieved through surgical implantation of invasive devices, such as microelectrodes, or externally with the use of noninvasive devices.

Paroxysmal hemicrania
A rare primary headache of the TAC group characterized by frequent, unilateral attacks that may occur up to 40 times a day.

Pathogenesis
The abnormal biological and physiological mechanisms that are associated with the origin and development of a disease (in this case, headaches). It is often used interchangeably with the term "etiopathogenesis."

Pathophysiology
The sum of the physical and biological abnormalities that are associated with a disease (in this case, headaches).

Primary headache
A headache that is a condition on its own rather than the symptom of an underlying disease or condition.

Prodromal phase
A series of early signs or symptoms that usually manifest before the onset of an attack and that act as anticipatory signs.

Prophylactic treatment
A therapy that aims at preventing a condition altogether rather than dealing with it at its onset.

Secondary headache
A headache that is the result of an underlying disease that triggers pain-sensitive areas in the neck and head.

SUNCT/SUNA
Rare primary headaches of the TAC group characterized by sudden and extremely painful attacks lasting a very short time and accompanied by distinct autonomic symptoms.

Tension-type headache (TTH)
Though relatively mild, one of the most prevalent headache disorders due to its ubiquitousness.

Thunderclap headache
An explosive and sudden high-intensity headache of abrupt onset that can last from 1 hour up to 10 days. Can be either a primary, benign headache of idiopathic origins or a secondary headache associated with some life-threatening vascular disorders.

Trepanation
An ancient surgical procedure through which a hole was drilled in the patient's skull. It was wrongly thought to be a potential treatment for persistent headaches. Also known as trepanning.

Trigeminalautonomic cephalalgias (TACs)
A group of primary headaches characterized by recurring, intense pain and the strong involvement of the autonomic nervous system. TACs include cluster headache, paroxysmal hemicrania, SUNCT, SUNA, and hemicrania continua.

Trigeminal neuralgia
A primary headache characterized by chronic neuropathic pain that affects the trigeminal (fifth cranial) nerve.

Trigeminovascular system
An important pain-signaling pathway of the brain consisting of nerve fibers of the head, neck, and face and the blood vessels they innervate. Its activation is known to be involved in the generation of the pain and symptoms that characterize many primary headaches.

Trigger
Factors or circumstances that are known to be able to flare up a headache attack. They tend to be consistent in each patient and include certain foods, lack of sleep, stress, and specific odors, among others.

Triptans
A category of medications of the tryptamine family used as abortive therapy in the treatment of migraines and cluster headaches. They act as agonists for 5-hydroxytryptamine (5-HT) receptors.

Directory of Resources

WEBSITES AND ORGANIZATIONS

American Academy of Neurology (AAN)
https://www.aan.com
Phone: (800) 879-1960 or (612) 928-6000 (International)
Fax: 612-454-2746
memberservices@aan.com
201 Chicago Avenue
Minneapolis, MN 55415
USA
The American Academy of Neurology (AAN) strives to promote the highest-quality patient-centered neurologic care and enhance member career satisfaction.

American Headache Society (AHS)
https://americanheadachesociety.org
Phone: 856-423-0043
Fax: 856-423-0082
ahshq@talley.com
19 Mantua Rd
Mount Royal, NJ 08061
USA
The American Headache Society (AHS) is a professional society of health-care providers dedicated to the study and treatment of headache and face pain. Its mission is to promote the exchange of information and ideas concerning the causes and treatments of headache and related painful disorders and ultimately to improve the care and lives of people living with headache disorders.

American Migraine Foundation
https://americanmigrainefoundation.org
Phone: 856-423-0043
Fax: 856-423-0082
amf@talley.com
19 Mantua Rd.
Mount Royal, NJ 08061
USA
American Migraine Foundation's mission is to mobilize a community for patient support and advocacy, as well as drive and support impactful research that translates into advances for patients with migraine and other disabling diseases that cause severe head pain.

Clusterbusters
https://clusterbusters.org
Clusterbusters, Inc.
PO Box 574
Lombard, IL 60148
USA
Clusterbusters is a nonprofit organization that supports research for better treatments and a cure while advocating to improve the lives of those struggling with cluster headaches.

European Headache Federation (EHF)
https://ehf-org.org
Phone: +49 3641 31 16 365 (Jutta Vach)
Phone: +49 3641 31 16 400 (Franziska Srp-Cappello)
Fax: +49 3641 31 16 243
ehf@conventus.de
Carl-Pulfrich-Str.1
07745 Jena
Germany
The European Headache Federation (EHF) is a nonprofit organization that dedicates its efforts to improving awareness of headache disorders and their impact among governments, health-care providers, and consumers across Europe.

European Migraine & Headache Alliance (EMH)
https://www.emhalliance.org
communications@emhalliance.org
Rue d'Egmont 11
1000 Brussels
Belgium

The European Migraine & Headache Alliance (EHMA) is a nonprofit umbrella organization that includes over 30 patient associations for migraine, cluster headache, trigeminal neuralgia, and other headache diseases, across Europe.

Facial Pain Association (FPA)
https://fpa-support.org
Phone: 1-800-923-3608 or 1-352-384-3600
info@tna-support.org
4600 SW 34th Street, #141592
Gainesville, FL 32614
USA
The Facial Pain Association (FPA), formerly known as the Trigeminal Neuralgia Association (TNA), is the world's leading resource for information and health-care guidance for all people suffering from neuropathic facial pain and trigeminal neuralgia. Patients, their loved ones, and health-care professionals can benefit from its programs of education, personal support, and advocacy efforts.

International Headache Society (IHS)
https://ihs-headache.org/en
carol.taylor@i-h-s.org
International Headache Society
4th Floor, Mitre House
44–46 Fleet Street
London, EC4Y 1BN.
United Kingdom
The IHS is an international professional organization working with others for the benefit of people affected by headache disorders. Its purpose is to advance headache science, education, and management and to promote headache awareness worldwide.

International Headache Society—Global Patient Advocacy Coalition (IHS-GPAC)
https://ihs-gpac.org/
info@ihs-gpac.org
IHS-GPAC
4th Floor, Mitre House
44–46 Fleet Street
London, EC4Y 1BN
United Kingdom
The International Headache Society—Global Patient Advocacy Coalition (IHS-GPAC) is a collective of the most influential voices in migraine

research, advocacy, and patient education formed to unify patient advocacies around the world and leverage collective resources to drive meaningful change in migraine patient care. Its aim is to reach health-care providers, policy makers, people living with migraine, and those around them in order to drive recognition of the impact of migraine on the individual and society.

Migraine Research Foundation (MRF)
https://migraineresearchfoundation.org/
info@migraineresearchfoundation.org
300 East 75th Street
Suite 3K
New York, NY 10021
USA
The Migraine Research Foundation (MRF) is a charity that raises money to award grants to researchers from around the world who are working to discover the causes, improve the treatments, and find a cure for migraine.

National Headache Foundation
https://headaches.org/
Phone: 312-274-2650
Toll-Free: 888-NHF-5552 (888-643-5552)
info@headaches.org
National Headache Foundation
820 N. Orleans
Suite 201
Chicago, IL 60610-3131
USA
The National Headache Foundation's mission is to further awareness of headache and migraine as legitimate neurobiological diseases. It serves as a resource for headache patients, doctors, and other health professionals.

BOOKS AND DOCUMENTS

Diamond, Seymour. *Headache and migraine biology and management.* Elsevier AP, 2015.

Eadie, Mervyn J. *Headache: Through the centuries.* Oxford University Press, 2012.

Foxhall, K. *Migraine: A history.* Johns Hopkins University Press; 2019.

Hattle, Ashley S. *Cluster headaches attack: A guide to surviving one of the most painful conditions known to man: For patients, supporters, & health care professionals.* BookBaby, 2017.

International Headache Society (IHS) (2020). International classification of orofacial pain, 1st edition (ICOP). *Cephalalgia: An International Journal of Headache, 40*(2), 129–221. https://doi.org/10.1177/0333102419893823

International Headache Society (2021). *The international classification of headache disorders* (3rd ed.). https://ichd-3.org/wp-content/uploads/2018/01/The-International-Classification-of-Headache-Disorders-3rd-Edition-2018.pdf

Leone, Massimo, and Arne May (2020). *Cluster headache and other trigeminal autonomic cephalgias.* Springer.

Steiner, T. (2005). Lifting the burden: The global campaign to reduce the burden of headache worldwide. *Journal of Headache and Pain, 6*(5), 373–377. https://doi: 10.1007/s10194-005-0241-7

Stovner, L. J., Hagen, K., Jensen, R., Katsarava, Z., Lipton, R., Scher, A., Steiner, T., et al. (2007). The global burden of headache: A documentation of headache prevalence and disability worldwide. *Cephalalgia: An International Journal of Headache, 27*(3), 193–210. https://doi.org/10.1111/j.1468-2982.2007.01288.x

World Health Organization (2011). *Atlas of headache disorders and resources in the world 2011.* WHO. https://apps.who.int/iris/handle/10665/44571

Bibliography

Aamodt, A. H., Stovner, L. J., Langhammer, A., Hagen, K., & Zwart, J. A. (2007). Is headache related to asthma, hay fever, and chronic bronchitis? The Head-HUNT Study. *Headache, 47*(2), 204–212. https://doi.org/10.1111/j.1526-4610.2006.00597.x

Adeney, K. L., & Williams, M. A. (2006). Migraine headaches and pre-eclampsia: An epidemiologic review. *Headache, 46*(5), 794–803. https://doi.org/10.1111/j.1526-4610.2006.00432.x

Agosti, R. (2018). Migraine burden of disease: From the patient's experience to a socio-economic view. *Headache, 58 Suppl 1*, 17–32. https://doi.org/10.1111/head.13301

Alstadhaug, K. B., Ofte, H. K., & Kristoffersen, E. S. (2017). Preventing and treating medication overuse headache. *Pain Reports, 2*(4), e612. https://doi.org/10.1097/PR9.0000000000000612

Antonaci, F., Nappi, G., Galli, F., Manzoni, G., Calabresi, P., & Costa, A. (2011). Migraine and psychiatric comorbidity: A review of clinical findings. *The Journal of Headache and Pain, 12*(2), 115–125. https://doi: 10.1007/s10194-010-0282-4

Bajaj, J., & Munakomi, S. (2020). Migraine surgical interventions. [Updated 2020 Jul 4]. In *StatPearls* [Internet]. Treasure Island, FL: StatPearls Publishing. Retrieved from https://www.ncbi.nlm.nih.gov/books/NBK525950

Bandarian-Balooch, S., Martin, P., McNally, B., Brunelli, A., & Mackenzie, S. (2017). Electronic-Diary for recording headaches, triggers, and medication use: Development and evaluation. *Headache, 57*(10), 1551–1569. https://doi: 10.1111/head.13184

Baron, E. P. (2018). Medicinal properties of cannabinoids, terpenes, and flavonoids in cannabis, and benefits in migraine, headache, and pain: An update on current evidence and cannabis science. *Headache, 58*(7), 1139–1186. https://doi.org/10.1111/head.13345

Becker, W. J. (2013). Cluster headache: Conventional pharmacological management. *Headache, 53*(7), 1191–1196. https://doi.org/10.1111/head.12145

Belcastro, V., Striano, P., Kasteleijn-Nolst Trenité, D. G., Villa, M. P., & Parisi, P. (2011). Migralepsy, hemicrania epileptica, post-ictal headache and "ictal epileptic headache": A proposal for terminology and classification revision. *The Journal of Headache and Pain, 12*(3), 289–294. https://doi.org/10.1007/s10194-011-0318-4

Bendtsen, L. (2000). Central sensitization in tension-type headache: Possible pathophysiological mechanisms. *Cephalalgia, 20*(5), 486–508. https://doi.org/10.1046/j.1468-2982.2000.00070.x

Bendtsen, L. (2009). Drug and nondrug treatment in tension-type headache. *Therapeutic Advances in Neurological Disorders, 2*(3), 155–161. https://doi.org/10.1177/1756285609102328

Benoliel, R. (2012). Trigeminal autonomic cephalgias. *British Journal of Pain, 6*(3), 106–123. https://doi.org/10.1177/2049463712456355

Brna, P., Dooley, J., Gordon, K., & Dewan, T. (2005). The prognosis of childhood headache: A 20-year follow-up. *Archives of Pediatrics & Adolescent Medicine, 159*(12), 1157–1160. https://doi.org/10.1001/archpedi.159.12.1157

Burstein, R., Noseda, R., & Borsook, D. (2015). Migraine: Multiple processes, complex pathophysiology. *The Journal of Neuroscience, 35*(17), 6619–6629. https://doi.org/10.1523/JNEUROSCI.0373-15.2015

Burton, W. N., Landy, S. H., Downs, K. E., & Runken, M. C. (2009). The impact of migraine and the effect of migraine treatment on workplace productivity in the United States and suggestions for future research. *Mayo Clinic Proceedings, 84*(5), 436–445. Retrieved from https://www.ncbi.nlm.nih.gov/pmc/articles/PMC2676126/

Buse, D. C., Fanning, K. M., Reed, M. L., Murray, S., Dumas, P. K., Adams, A. M., & Lipton, R. B. (2019). Life with migraine: Effects on relationships, career, and finances from the Chronic Migraine Epidemiology and Outcomes (CaMEO) study. *Headache, 59*(8), 1286–1299. https://doi.org/10.1111/head.13613

Buse, D. C., Reed, M. L., Fanning, K. M., Bostic, R., Dodick, D. W., Schwedt, T. J., Munjal, S., et al. (2020). Comorbid and co-occurring conditions in migraine and associated risk of increasing headache pain intensity and headache frequency: Results of the Migraine in America Symptoms and Treatment (MAST) study. *The Journal of Headache and Pain, 21*(1), 23. https://doi.org/10.1186/s10194-020-1084-y

Buse, D. C., Scher, A. I., Dodick, D. W., Reed, M. L., Fanning, K. M., Manack Adams, A., & Lipton, R. B. (2016). Impact of migraine on the family: Perspectives of people with migraine and their spouse/domestic partner in the CaMEO study. *Mayo Clinic Proceedings*, S0025-6196(16)00126-9. https://doi.org/10.1016/j.mayocp.2016.02.013

Calixto, J. B. (2000). Efficacy, safety, quality control, marketing and regulatory guidelines for herbal medicines (phytotherapeutic agents). *Brazilian Journal of Medical and Biological Research*, *33*(2), 179–189. https://doi.org/10.1590/s0100-879x2000000200004

Charles, A., & Brennan, K. (2009). Cortical spreading depression: New insights and persistent questions. *Cephalalgia*, *29*(10), 1115–1124. https://doi.org/10.1111/j.1468-2982.2009.01983.x

Chowdhury, D. (2012). Tension type headache. *Annals of Indian Academy of Neurology*, *15*(Suppl. 1), S83–S88. https://doi.org/10.4103/0972-2327.100023

Cohen, A. (2014). Trigeminal autonomic cephalalgias: A diagnostic and therapeutic overview. *Advances in Clinical Neuroscience & Rehabilitation Online*, *14*(4), 12–15.

Cohen, A. S., Matharu, M. S., & Goadsby, P. J. (2006). Short-lasting unilateral neuralgiform headache attacks with conjunctival injection and tearing (SUNCT) or cranial autonomic features (SUNA): A prospective clinical study of SUNCT and SUNA. *Brain*, *129*(Pt. 10), 2746–2760. https://doi.org/10.1093/brain/awl202

Cozzolino, O., Marchese, M., Trovato, F., Pracucci, E., Ratto, G. M., Buzzi, M. G., Sicca, F., et al. (2018). Understanding spreading depression from headache to sudden unexpected death. *Frontiers in Neurology*, *9*, 19. https://doi.org/10.3389/fneur.2018.00019

Cutrer, M. F., & O'Donnell, A. (2004). Chapter 19: Pathophysiology of headaches. In C. Warfield & Z. Bajwa (Eds.). *Principles and practice of pain medicine* (2nd ed.). New York: McGraw Hill.

Demaagd, G. (2008a). The pharmacological management of migraine, part 1: Overview and abortive therapy. *P & T*, *33*(7), 404–416.

Demaagd, G. (2008b). The pharmacological management of migraine, part 2: Preventative therapy. *P & T*, *33*(8), 480–487.

Din, L., & Lui, F. (2020). Butterbur. [Updated 2020 Jul 6]. In *StatPearls* [Internet]. Treasure Island, FL: StatPearls Publishing. Retrieved from https://www.ncbi.nlm.nih.gov/books/NBK537160

Dodick, D. W., Loder, E. W., Manack Adams, A., Buse, D. C., Fanning, K. M., Reed, M. L., & Lipton, R. B. (2016). Assessing barriers to chronic migraine consultation, diagnosis, and treatment: Results from the Chronic Migraine Epidemiology and Outcomes (CaMEO) study. *Headache*, *56*(5), 821–834. https://doi.org/10.1111/head.12774

Eadie, M. J. (2012). Chronic paroxysmal hemicrania. In *Headache: Through the centuries* (pp. 222–224). New York: Oxford University Press.

Edgunlu, T., & Celik, S. (2017). Genetic aspect of headache. In *Current perspectives on less-known aspects of headache*. Retrieved from https://

www.intechopen.com/books/current-perspectives-on-less-known
-aspects-of-headache/genetic-aspect-of-headache

Ferrante, E., Tassorelli, C., Rossi, P., Lisotto, C., & Nappi, G. (2011). Focus on the management of thunderclap headache: From nosography to treatment. *The Journal of Headache and Pain, 12*(2), 251–258. https://doi.org/10.1007/s10194-011-0302-z

Fletcher, J. (2015). Why cluster headaches are called "suicide headaches." *Journal of Neurology & Stroke, 3*(3). https://doi.org/10.15406/jnsk.2015.03.00092

Foxhall, K. (2018, March 12). Migraine myth: Drilling holes in the skull was never a cure—but it was long thought to be. *The Independent.* Retrieved from https://www.independent.co.uk/life-style/health-and-families/migraine-cure-trepanning-trepanation-drill-holes-skull-ancient-humans-stone-age-a8243381.html

Foxhall, K. (2019a). "The pain was very much relieved and she slept": Gender and patienthood in the nineteenth century. In *Migraine: A history* [Internet]. Baltimore, MD: Johns Hopkins University Press. Retrieved from https://www.ncbi.nlm.nih.gov/books/NBK544085

Foxhall, K. (2019b). "Take housleeke, and garden wormes": Migraine medicine in the early modern household. In *Migraine: A history* [Internet]. Baltimore, MD: Johns Hopkins University Press. Retrieved from https://www.ncbi.nlm.nih.gov/books/NBK544091

Gambeta, E., Chichorro, J. G., & Zamponi, G. W. (2020). Trigeminal neuralgia: An overview from pathophysiology to pharmacological treatments. *Molecular Pain, 16*, 1744806920901890. https://doi.org/10.1177/1744806920901890

GBD 2016 Headache Collaborators. (2018). Global, regional, and national burden of migraine and tension-type headache, 1990–2016: A systematic analysis for the Global Burden of Disease Study 2016. *The Lancet, 17*(11), 954–976. https://doi.org/10.1016/S1474-4422(18)30322-3

Goadsby, P. J. (2009). The vascular theory of migraine--a great story wrecked by the facts. *Brain, 132*(Pt. 1), 6–7. https://doi.org/10.1093/brain/awn321

Goadsby, P. J. (2012). Pathophysiology of migraine. *Annals of Indian Academy of Neurology, 15*(Suppl. 1), S15–S22. https://doi.org/10.4103/0972-2327.99993

Goldberg, L. D. (2005). The cost of migraine and its treatment. *The American Journal of Managed Care, 11*(2 Suppl.), S62–S67.

Heckman, B. D., & Holroyd, K. A. (2006). Tension-type headache and psychiatric comorbidity. *Current Pain and Headache Reports, 10*(6), 439–447. https://doi.org/10.1007/s11916-006-0075-2

Holroyd, K. A., Stensland, M., Lipchik, G. L., Hill, K. R., O'Donnell, F. S., & Cordingley, G. (2000). Psychosocial correlates and impact of

chronic tension-type headaches. *Headache, 40*(1), 3–16. https://doi
.org/10.1046/j.1526-4610.2000.00001.x

International Association for the Study of Pain. (2011). *Epidemiology of
headache.* Retrieved from https://s3.amazonaws.com/rdcms-iasp
/files/production/public/Content/ContentFolders/GlobalYearAgainst
Pain2/HeadacheFactSheets/1-Epidemiology.pdf

Joshi, S., Rizzoli, P., & Loder, E. (2017). The comorbidity burden of patients
with cluster headache: A population-based study. *The Journal of Headache and Pain, 18*(1), 76. https://doi.org/10.1186/s10194-017-0785-3

Kacperski, J., Kabbouche, M. A., O'Brien, H. L., & Weberding, J. L. (2016).
The optimal management of headaches in children and adolescents. *Therapeutic Advances in Neurological Disorders, 9*(1), 53–68.
https://doi.org/10.1177/1756285615616586

Kapoor, S. (2013). Headache attributed to cranial or cervical vascular disorders. *Current Pain and Headache Reports, 17*(5), 334. https://doi
.org/10.1007/s11916-013-0334-y

Koehler, P. J., & Boes, C. J. (2010). A history of non-drug treatment in headache, particularly migraine. *Brain, 133*(Pt. 8), 2489–2500. https://
doi:10.1093/brain/awq170

Kreling, G., de Almeida Neto, N. R., & dos Santos Neto, P. J. (2017).
Migrainous infarction: A rare and often overlooked diagnosis. *Autopsy & Case Reports, 7*(2), 61–68. https://doi.org/10.4322
/acr.2017.018

Kristoffersen, E. S., & Lundqvist, C. (2014). Medication-overuse headache:
Epidemiology, diagnosis and treatment. *Therapeutic Advances in
Drug Safety, 5*(2), 87–99. https://doi.org/10.1177/2042098614522683

Kroon Van Diest, A. M., Ernst, M. M., Slater, S., & Powers, S. W. (2017).
Similarities and differences between migraine in children and
adults: Presentation, disability, and response to treatment. *Current
Pain and Headache Reports, 21*(12), 48. https://doi.org/10.1007
/s11916-017-0648-2

Lambru, G., & Matharu, M. S. (2012). Trigeminal autonomic cephalalgias:
A review of recent diagnostic, therapeutic and pathophysiological
developments. *Annals of Indian Academy of Neurology, 15*(Suppl.
1), S51–S61. https://doi.org/10.4103/0972-2327.100007

Lambru, G., & Matharu, M. S. (2013). SUNCT and SUNA: Medical and
surgical treatments. *Neurological Sciences, 34*(Suppl. 1), S75–S81.
https://doi.org/10.1007/s10072-013-1366-0

Leonardi, M., & Raggi, A. (2019). A narrative review on the burden of migraine:
When the burden is the impact on people's life. *The Journal of Headache and Pain, 20*(1), 41. https://doi.org/10.1186/s10194-019-0993-0

Leone, M., Franzini, A., Proietti Cecchini, A., Broggi, G., & Bussone, G.
(2010). Hypothalamic deep brain stimulation in the treatment of

chronic cluster headache. *Therapeutic Advances In Neurological Disorders, 3*(3), 187–195. https://doi:10.1177/1756285610370722

Lipton, R. B., Bigal, M. E., Ashina, S., Burstein, R., Silberstein, S., Reed, M. L., Serrano, D., et al. (2008). Cutaneous allodynia in the migraine population. *Annals of Neurology, 63*(2), 148–158. https://doi.org /10.1002/ana.21211

Lipton, R. B., Buse, D. C., Hall, C. B., Tennen, H., Defreitas, T. A., Borkowski, T. M., Grosberg, B. M., et al. (2014). Reduction in perceived stress as a migraine trigger: Testing the "let-down headache" hypothesis. *Neurology, 82*(16), 1395–1401. https://doi.org/10.1212/WNL .0000000000000332

Loder, E., & Rizzoli, P. (2008). Tension-type headache. *BMJ, 336*(7635), 88–92. https://doi.org/10.1136/bmj.39412.705868.AD

Maghbooli, M., Golipour, F., Moghimi Esfandabadi, A., & Yousefi, M. (2014). Comparison between the efficacy of ginger and sumatriptan in the ablative treatment of the common migraine. *Phytotherapy Research: PTR, 28*(3), 412–415. https://doi.org/10.1002/ptr.4996

Magiorkinis, E., Diamantis, A., Mitsikostas, D. D., & Androutsos, G. (2009). Headaches in antiquity and during the early scientific era. *Journal of Neurology, 256*(8), 1215–1220. https://doi.org/10.1007 /s00415-009-5085-7

Malone, C. D., Bhowmick, A., & Wachholtz, A. B. (2015). Migraine: Treatments, comorbidities, and quality of life, in the USA. *Journal of Pain Research, 8*: 537–547. https://doi.org/10.2147/JPR.S88207

Manzoni, G., & Stovner, L. (2010). Epidemiology of headache. In *Handbook of clinical neurology* (pp. 3–22). https://doi: 10.1016/s0072-9752(10) 97001-2

Martelletti, P., Schwedt, T. J., Lanteri-Minet, M., Quintana, R., Carboni, V., Diener, H. C., Ruiz de la Torre, E., et al. (2018). My Migraine Voice survey: A global study of disease burden among individuals with migraine for whom preventive treatments have failed. *The Journal of Headache and Pain, 19*(1), 115. https://doi.org/10.1186/s10194 -018-0946-z

Marukatat, C., Phiphopthatsanee, N., Nimnuan, C., Srikiatkhachorn, A., & Wang, S. J. (2020, January 25). Epidemiology of headache. *Medlink*. Retrieved from https://www.medlink.com/index.php/article /epidemiology_of_headache

Mason, B. N., & Russo, A. F. (2018). Vascular contributions to migraine: Time to revisit? *Frontiers in Cellular Neuroscience, 12*, 233. https:// doi.org/10.3389/fncel.2018.00233

May, A., Leone, M., Afra, J., Linde, M., Sándor, P. S., Evers, S., Goadsby, P. J., et al. (2006). EFNS guidelines on the treatment of cluster headache and other trigeminal-autonomic cephalalgias. *European Journal of Neurology, 13*(10), 1066–1077. https://doi.org/10.1111/j.1468-1331.2006.01566.x

Mazzei, R., De Marco, E. V., Gallo, O., & Tagarelli, G. (2018). Italian folk plant-based remedies to heal headache (XIX-XX century). *Journal of Ethnopharmacology, 210,* 417–433. https://doi.org/10.1016/j .jep.2017.09.005

McAllister, P. (2018, October). Headache horizons: Tuning in to psychedelics for treatment of suicide headaches. *Practical Neurology.* Retrieved from https://practicalneurology.com/articles/2018-oct /headache-horizons-tuning-in-to-psychedelics-for-treatment-of -suicide-headaches

Millea, P. J., & Brodie, J. J. (2002). Tension-type headache. *American Family Physician, 66*(5), 797–804.

Minen, M. T., Begasse De Dhaem, O., Kroon Van Diest, A., Powers, S., Schwedt, T. J., Lipton, R., & Silbersweig, D. (2016). Migraine and its psychiatric comorbidities. *Journal of Neurology, Neurosurgery, and Psychiatry, 87*(7), 741–749.

Modi, S., & Lowder, D. M. (2006). Medications for migraine prophylaxis. *American Family Physician, 73*(1), 72–78.

National Clinical Guideline Centre (UK). (2012). *Headaches: Diagnosis and management of headaches in young people and adults* [Internet]. Clinical Guidelines 150. London: Royal College of Physicians. Retrieved from https://www.ncbi.nlm.nih.gov/books/NBK327511.

Nebel, R. A. (2019). Assessing and treating migraine in women and men. *Practical Pain Management, 19*(1), 45-47.

Nowaczewska, M., Wiciński, M., Osiński, S., & Kaźmierczak, H. (2020). The role of Vitamin D in primary headache–from potential mechanism to treatment. *Nutrients, 12*(1), 243. https://doi.org/10.3390 /nu12010243

Obermann, M. (2010). Treatment options in trigeminal neuralgia. *Therapeutic Advances in Neurological Disorders, 3*(2), 107–115. https:// doi.org/10.1177/1756285609359317

Obrenovitch, T., & Dreier, J. (2021). *Migraine with aura.* Migraine Trust. Retrieved from https://www.migrainetrust.org/about-migraine/types -of-migraine/migraine-with-aura

Osman, C., & Bahra, A. (2018). Paroxysmal hemicrania. *Annals of Indian Academy of Neurology, 21*(Suppl. 1), S16–S22. https://doi.org/10.4103 /aian.AIAN_317_17

Pareja, J. A., & Sjaastad, O. (2010). Primary stabbing headache. *Handbook of Clinical Neurology, 97,* 453–457. https://doi.org/10.1016/S0072 -9752(10)97039-5

Peterlin, B. L., Gupta, S., Ward, T. N., & Macgregor, A. (2011). Sex matters: Evaluating sex and gender in migraine and headache research. *Headache, 51*(6), 839–842. https://doi.org/10.1111/j.1526-4610.2011.01900.x

Pilitsis, J., & Khazen, O. (2021). *Trigeminal neuralgia—causes, symptoms and treatments.* American Association of Neurological Surgeons.

Retrieved from https://www.aans.org/Patients/Neurosurgical -Conditions-and-Treatments/Trigeminal-Neuralgia

Prakash, S., & Patel, P. (2017). Hemicrania continua: Clinical review, diagnosis and management. *Journal of Pain Research*, *10*, 1493–1509. https://doi.org/10.2147/JPR.S128472

Puledda, F., & Shields, K. (2018). Non-Pharmacological approaches for migraine. *Neurotherapeutics*, *15*(2), 336–345. https://doi.org/10.1007 /s13311-018-0623-6

Rasmussen, B. K., Jensen, R., Schroll, M., & Olesen, J. (1991). Epidemiology of headache in a general population--a prevalence study. *Journal of Clinical Epidemiology*, *44*(11), 1147–1157. https://doi.org/10.1016 /0895-4356(91)90147-2

Ruau, D., Liu, L. Y., Clark, J. D., Angst, M. S., & Butte, A. J. (2012). Sex differences in reported pain across 11,000 patients captured in electronic medical records. *The Journal of Pain*, *13*(3), 228–234. https:// doi.org/10.1016/j.jpain.2011.11.002

Rules, T. (2014, November 11). *I have the worst headache in the world*. Vice. Retrieved from https://www.vice.com/en/article/vdpnmy/the-worst -headache-in-the-world-876

Sabalys, G., Juodzbalys, G., & Wang, H. L. (2013). Aetiology and pathogenesis of trigeminal neuralgia: A comprehensive review. *Journal of Oral & Maxillofacial Research*, *3*(4), e2. https://doi.org/10.5037/jomr.2012.3402

Scher, A. I., Midgette, L. A., & Lipton, R. B. (2008). Risk factors for headache chronification. *Headache*, *48*(1), 16–25. https://doi.org/10.1111 /j.1526-4610.2007.00970.x

Sewell, R. A., Halpern, J. H., & Pope, H. G., Jr. (2006). Response of cluster headache to psilocybin and LSD. *Neurology*, *66*(12), 1920–1922. https://doi.org/10.1212/01.wnl.0000219761.05466.43

Shah, U. H., & Kalra, V. (2009). Pediatric migraine. *International Journal of Pediatrics*, *2009*, 424192. https://doi.org/10.1155/2009/424192

Sheftell, F., & Bigal, M. (2004). Headache and psychiatric comorbidity. *Psychiatric Times*, *21*(12). Retrieved from https://www.psychiatrictimes .com/view/headache-and-psychiatric-comorbidity

Shevel E. (2011). The extracranial vascular theory of migraine: An artificial controversy. *Journal of Neural Transmission*, *118*(4), 525–530. https://doi.org/10.1007/s00702-010-0517-1

Sinclair, A. J., Sturrock, A., Davies, B., & Matharu, M. (2015). Headache management: Pharmacological approaches. *Practical Neurology*, *15*(6), 411–423. https://doi.org/10.1136/practneurol-2015-001167

Song, T. J., Lee, M. J., Choi, Y. J., Kim, B. K., Chung, P. W., Park, J. W., Chu, M. K., et al. (2019). Differences in characteristics and comorbidity of cluster headache according to the presence of migraine. *Journal of Clinical Neurology, 15*(3), 334–338. https://doi.org/10.3988/jcn.2019.15.3.334

Starling, A. J., Hoffman-Snyder, C., Halker, R. B., Wellik, K. E., Vargas, B. B., Dodick, D. W., Demaerschalk, B. M., et al. (2011). Risk of development of medication overuse headache with nonsteroidal anti-inflammatory drug therapy for migraine: A critically appraised topic. *The Neurologist, 17*(5), 297–299. https://doi.org/10.1097/NRL.0b013e31822d109c

Stern, S., Cifu, A., & Altkorn, D. (2014). *Symptom to diagnosis: An evidence-based guide* (3rd ed.). New York: McGraw-Hill.

Straube, A., & Andreou, A. (2019). Primary headaches during lifespan. *The Journal of Headache and Pain, 20*(1), 35. https://doi.org/10.1186/s10194-019-0985-0

Sun-Edelstein, C., & Mauskop, A. (2011). Alternative headache treatments: Nutraceuticals, behavioral and physical treatments. *Headache, 51*(3), 469–483. https://doi.org/10.1111/j.1526-4610.2011.01846.x

Tepper, S., & Johnstone, M. (2018). Breath-powered sumatriptan dry nasal powder: An intranasal medication delivery system for acute treatment of migraine. *Medical Devices: Evidence and Research, 11*, 147–156. https://doi.org/10.2147/mder.s130900

Trejo-Gabriel-Galan, J. M., Aicua-Rapún, I., Cubo-Delgado, E., & Velasco-Bernal, C. (2018). Suicide in primary headaches in 48 countries: A physician-survey based study. *Cephalalgia, 38*(4), 798–803. https://doi.org/10.1177/0333102417714477

Verhagen, A. P., Damen, L., Berger, M. Y., Passchier, J., & Koes, B. W. (2009). Behavioral treatments of chronic tension-type headache in adults: Are they beneficial? *CNS Neuroscience & Therapeutics, 15*(2), 183–205. https://doi.org/10.1111/j.1755-5949.2009.00077.x

Vinciguerra, L., Cantone, M., Lanza, G., Bramanti, A., Santalucia, P., Puglisi, V., Pennisi, G., et al. (2019). Migrainous infarction and cerebral vasospasm: Case report and literature review. *Journal of Pain Research, 12*, 2941–2950. https://doi.org/10.2147/JPR.S209485

Wang, S. J., Chen, P. K., & Fuh, J. L. (2010). Comorbidities of migraine. *Frontiers in Neurology, 1*, 16. https://doi.org/10.3389/fneur.2010.00016

Waters, W. (1971). Migraine: Intelligence, social class, and familial prevalence. *BMJ, 2*(5753), 77–81. https://doi.org/10.1136/bmj.2.5753.77

Wider, B., Pittler, M. H., & Ernst, E. (2004). Feverfew for preventing migraine. *Cochrane Database of Systematic Reviews*, (1), CD002286. Retrieved from https://www.cochrane.org/CD002286/feverfew-preventing-migraine#

World Health Organization. (2011). *Atlas of headache disorders and resources in the world 2011*. Geneva: WHO.

World Health Organization. (2016, April 8). *Headache disorders—key facts.* Retrieved from https://www.who.int/news-room/fact-sheets/detail /headache-disorders

Wu, J., & Wang, S. J. (2019, May 22). Headache attributed to head trauma. *Medlink.* Retrieved from https://www.medlink.com/articles/headache -attributed-to-head-trauma

Young, W. B., Park, J. E., Tian, I. X., & Kempner, J. (2013). The stigma of migraine. *PloS One, 8*(1), e54074. https://doi.org/10.1371/journal .pone.0054074

Index

About the Author

Dr. Claudio Butticè, Pharm.D., is a former clinical and hospital pharmacist who worked for several public hospitals in Italy as well as for the humanitarian NGO Emergency. He is now an accomplished book author who has written on topics such as medicine, technology, world poverty, human rights, and science. His latest book is *Universal Health Care* (Greenwood, 2019). A data analyst and freelance journalist as well, many of his articles have been published in magazines such as *Cracked, The Elephant, Digital Journal, The Ring of Fire,* and *Business Insider.* Dr. Butticè has also published pharmacology and psychology papers in several clinical journals and works as a medical consultant and advisor for many companies across the globe.